Clinicians' Guides to Radionuclide Hybrid Imaging

PET/CT

W0050725

Series Editors

Jamshed B. Bomanji
London, UK

Gopinath Gnanasegaran
London, UK

Stefano Fanti
Bologna, Italy

Homer A. Macapinlac
Houston, Texas, USA

More information about this series at http://www.springer.com/series/13803

Yong Du
Editor

PET/CT in Colorectal Cancer

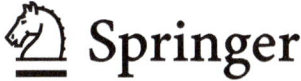

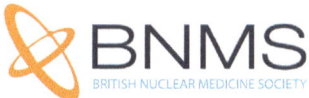

Editor
Yong Du
Department of Nuclear Medicine and PET/CT
Royal Marsden NHS Foundation Trust
London
United Kingdom

ISSN 2367-2439   ISSN 2367-2447   (electronic)
Clinicians' Guides to Radionuclide Hybrid Imaging - PET/CT
ISBN 978-3-319-54836-4   ISBN 978-3-319-54837-1   (eBook)
DOI 10.1007/978-3-319-54837-1

Library of Congress Control Number: 2017940858

Printed on acid-free paper

This Springer imprint is published by Springer Nature
The registered company is Springer International Publishing AG
The registered company address is: Gewerbestrasse 11, 6330 Cham, Switzerland

PET/CT series is dedicated to Prof Ignac Fogelman, Dr Muriel Buxton-Thomas and Prof Ajit K Padhy

Foreword

Clear and concise clinical indications for PET/CT in the management of the oncology patient are presented in this series of 15 separate booklets.

The impact on better staging, tailored management and specific treatment of the patient with cancer has been achieved with the advent of this multimodality imaging technology. Early and accurate diagnosis will always pay, and clear information can be gathered with PET/CT on treatment responses. Prognostic information is gathered and can further guide additional therapeutic options.

It is a fortunate coincidence that PET/CT was able to derive great benefit from radionuclide-labelled probes, which deliver good and often excellent target to non-target signals. Whilst labelled glucose remains the cornerstone for the clinical benefit achieved, a number of recent probes are definitely adding benefit. PET/CT is hence an evolving technology, extending its applications and indications. Significant advances in the instrumentation and data processing available have also contributed to this technology, which delivers high throughput and a wealth of data, with good patient tolerance and indeed patient and public acceptance. As an example, the role of PET/CT in the evaluation of cardiac disease is also covered, with emphasis on labelled rubidium and labelled glucose studies.

The novel probes of labelled choline; labelled peptides, such as DOTATATE; and, most recently, labelled PSMA (prostate-specific membrane antigen) have gained rapid clinical utility and acceptance, as significant PET/CT tools for the management of neuroendocrine disease and prostate cancer patients, notwithstanding all the advances achieved with other imaging modalities, such as MRI. Hence, a chapter reviewing novel PET tracers forms part of this series.

The oncological community has recognised the value of PET/CT and has delivered advanced diagnostic criteria for some of the most important indications for PET/CT. This includes the recent Deauville criteria for the classification of PET/CT patients with lymphoma—similar criteria are expected to develop for other malignancies, such as head and neck cancer, melanoma and pelvic malignancies. For completion, a separate section covers the role of PET/CT in radiotherapy planning, discussing the indications for planning biological tumour volumes in relevant cancers.

These booklets offer simple, rapid and concise guidelines on the utility of PET/CT in a range of oncological indications. They also deliver a rapid aide-memoire on the merits and appropriate indications for PET/CT in oncology.

London, UK   Peter J. Ell, FMedSci, DR HC, AΩA

Preface

Hybrid imaging with PET/CT and SPECT/CT combines the best of function and structure to provide accurate localisation, characterisation and diagnosis. There are extensive literature and evidence to support PET/CT, which have made significant impact in oncological imaging and management of patients with cancer. The evidence in favour of SPECT/CT especially in orthopaedic indications is evolving and increasing.

The *Clinicians' Guides to Radionuclide Hybrid Imaging* pocketbook series is specifically aimed at our referring clinicians, nuclear medicine/radiology doctors, radiographers/technologists and nurses who are routinely working in nuclear medicine and participate in multidisciplinary meetings. This series is the joint work of many friends and professionals from different nations who share a common dream and vision towards promoting and supporting nuclear medicine as a useful and important imaging speciality.

We want to thank all those people who have contributed to this work as advisors, authors and reviewers, without whom the book would not have been possible. We want to thank our members from the BNMS (British Nuclear Medicine Society, UK) for their encouragement and support, and we are extremely grateful to Dr Brian Nielly, Charlotte Weston, the BNMS Education Committee and the BNMS council members for their enthusiasm and trust.

Finally, we wish to extend particular gratitude to the industry for their continuous support towards education and training.

London, UK

Gopinath Gnanasegaran
Jamshed Bomanji

Acknowledgements

The series coordinators and editors would like to express their sincere gratitude to the members of the British Nuclear Medicine Society, patients, teachers, colleagues, students, the industry and the BNMS Education Committee members, for their continued support and inspiration:

Andy Bradley
Brent Drake
Francis Sundram
James Ballinger
Parthiban Arumugam
Rizwan Syed
Sai Han
Vineet Prakash

Contents

Contributors

Gayathri Anandappa GI Unit, The Royal Marsden Hospital NHS Foundation Trust, London, UK

Svetlana Balyasnikova The Royal Marsden NHS Foundation Trust, London, UK

Gina Brown Department of Radiology, The Royal Marsden NHS Foundation Trust, London, UK

Yong Du, M.B.B.S., M.Sc., Ph.D., F.R.C.P. Department of Nuclear Medicine and PET/CT, Royal Marsden NHS Foundation Trust, London, UK

Ajith Joy Department of Nuclear Medicine and PET/CT, KIMS-DDNMRC, Trivandrum, India

Chenggang Li Warrington and Halton Hospitals NHS Foundation Trust, Warrington, UK

Arun Sasikumar Department of Nuclear Medicine and PET/CT, KIMS-DDNMRC, Trivandrum, India

Vera Tudyka The Royal Marsden NHS Foundation Trust, London, UK
Croydon University Hospital, Croydon, UK

Introduction of Colorectal Cancer

1

Yong Du and Vera Tudyka

Contents

1.1 Introduction

Colorectal cancer, also called bowel cancer, is the third most common cancer in both males (14% of the male total) and females (11%) in the UK. In 2011, there were 41,581 new cases of bowel cancer in the UK. It is the second most common cause of cancer death in the UK, accounting for 10% of all deaths from cancer. The overall predicted 5-year survival rate is 59% for patients diagnosed with bowel cancer during

Y. Du (✉)
Department of Nuclear Medicine and PET/CT, Royal Marsden NHS Foundation Trust, London, UK
e-mail: yong.du@rmh.nhs.uk

V. Tudyka
The Royal Marsden NHS Foundation Trust, London, UK

Croydon University Hospital, Croydon, UK

© Springer International Publishing Switzerland 2017   1
Y. Du (ed.), *PET/CT in Colorectal Cancer*, Clinicians' Guides to Radionuclide
Hybrid Imaging - PET/CT, DOI 10.1007/978-3-319-54837-1_1

2010–2011 in England and Wales. Worldwide, it is also the third most common cancer, with more than 1,360,000 new cases diagnosed in 2012 (10% of the total) [1].

Bowel cancer mortality rates have decreased overall in the UK and Europe since the 1970s, likely owing to the earlier detection and improved treatment. Over the last decade, European age-standardised mortality rates have decreased by 15% in males and 12% in females with colorectal cancer. Nonetheless, the burden of the disease and mortality is still high, and further improvement in diagnostic accuracy including tumour-node-metastasis (TNM) staging and tumour biology characterisation remains essential for a better selection of treatment approaches by an experienced multidisciplinary expert team. In addition to conventional morphological imaging modalities such as CT, ultrasound and MRI, ¹⁸FDG-PET/CT plays instrumental roles in several areas critical for the optimal management of colorectal cancer.

1.2   Epidemiology

Highest incidence in North America, Australia, New Zealand and Western Europe

– Lowest incidence in Africa, Asia and South America
– Third most common malignancy in the Western world
– Second most common cause of cancer death in the Western world
– Male to female odds ratio for colon cancer 1.2:1
– Male to female odds ratio for rectal cancer 1.4:1
– Peak incidence age 60–70 years
– Lifetime risk 3–5%

Anatomic site

– Distribution: rectum 30% and colon 70%
– Distribution within the colon: caecum 16%, ascending colon 16%, hepatic flexure 7%, transverse colon 8%, splenic flexure 5%, descending colon 6% and sigmoid 42%
– Increasing incidence of right-sided cancers (less accessible for endoscopy, more flat lesions)
– Synchronous lesions: 4–5% [1, 2]

1.3   Causes/Risk Factors

– 95% sporadic, 5% familial/hereditary: familial adenomatous polyposis (FAP), Gardner syndrome, Peutz-Jeghers disease and hereditary nonpolyposis colorectal cancer (HNPCC)
– Alcohol and nicotine abuse
– Obesity
– 'Western' diet
– Age > 50 years

- Previous adenomas
- Previous colorectal malignancy
- Family history: 2–3 times increased risk if affected first-degree relative
- Inflammatory bowel disease (Crohn's disease, ulcerative colitis) [3, 4]

1.4   Clinical Presentation/Signs and Symptoms

About 30% of colorectal cancer is detected by screening of asymptomatic individuals. The majority of symptomatic patients presents with chronic symptoms. Emergent presentation occurs in about 16% of patients with colon cancer who present with mainly obstructive symptoms that warrant urgent surgery.

Most common chronic signs and symptoms are the following:

- Haematochezia or melena
- Abdominal pain
- Iron deficiency anaemia
- Change in bowel habit

Clinical manifestations correlate with the site of tumour location. Right-sided tumours rarely present as an obstructive emergency, as the right colon is relatively wide and faeces is still quite liquid in the proximal colon. Haematochezia is more common with distal tumours, while iron deficiency anaemia without haematochezia is more common with right-sided tumours. Abdominal pain is not typically associated with a specific tumour site within the colon or rectum. Abdominal pain might be a result of (partial) obstruction, ingrowth in surrounding organs or perforation with peritonitis. Rectal cancer can cause symptoms of tenesmus or rectal pain [3, 4].

1.5   Diagnosis

There are several modalities used in screening of colorectal cancer [5]:

- Faecal blood testing
- X-ray with barium enema
- Flexible sigmoidoscopy
- Colonoscopy
- CT colonography

Investigation for a (suspected) colorectal cancer should be appropriately measured to the patient's comorbidities and fitness. If a patient is too frail to undergo surgery or even (palliative) chemotherapy, the clinician should consider not to investigate any further at all [6]. Colonoscopy carries a risk of bleeding in 1.64/1000 and perforation in 0.85/1000, while CT has risks associated with the use of contrast agents and radiation [7, 8].

1.6   Faecal Occult Blood Testing (FOBT)

– Uses guaiac-based products or immunochemistry to test for microscopic blood in faeces
– Designed to be used at home
– Low sensitivity detection rate
– Low compliance rates of 60%
– Cost-effective

1.7   X-Ray with Barium Enema

– Low detection rate even for lesions >10 mm
– Impaired patient tolerance
– Grossly abandoned for screening for colorectal cancer, replaced by more accurate screening tools like colonoscopy and CT colonography

1.8   Flexible Sigmoidoscopy

– Covers the most common site of colorectal cancer (70% arise in the left colon)
– No sedation required
– No extensive bowel preparation needed
– Allows biopsies and polypectomies

1.9   Colonoscopy

– Visualises the complete colon up to the caecum
– Requires sedation in most cases
– Requires bowel preparation

Colonoscopy is regarded as the gold standard for diagnosing colorectal lesions. Colonoscopy visualises the complete colon and enables exclusion of polyps and other abnormalities. During colonoscopy, biopsies can be taken for histopathological confirmation of the diagnosis, and the lesion can be marked with tattoo, which enables identification of the site on a later stage during laparoscopic surgery. However, in certain cases colonoscopy might be incomplete. Patients might be intolerant to the procedure or might not be able to complete the mandatory bowel preparation or in case of obstruction colonoscopy might not be completed. In these cases CT colonography should be considered as an alternative [8, 9].

1.10   CT Colonography

CT colonography has a high sensitivity of 96%, equivalent to colonoscopy for lesions ≥10 mm. The disadvantage of this purely imaging tool is that it lacks the opportunity of taking biopsies or performing polypectomies. In up to 30% of cases, CT colonography will detect a lesion that demands a subsequent colonoscopy [10–14].

Table 1.1 Prognostic features of colorectal carcinoma

Good prognosis	Poor prognosis
T1 T2 T3a–b	T3c-d, T4
N0	N1–2
M0	M1
EMVI negative	EMVI positive
CRM negative	CRM involved

CT colonoscopy lacks accuracy in identifying lesions smaller than 5 mm. Therefore, CT colonography is less suitable for those patients with a high risk for carcinoma or adenoma as it might miss small lesions. However, CT colonography would be the preferred screening tool in elderly or frail patients who would not be able to undergo the consequences of complications of a colonoscopy such as perforation or bleeding that would need reintervention or surgery [10–14].

1.11 Staging Procedures/Investigations

Staging aims to stratify colorectal cancers into good and poor prognosis tumours. Poor prognosis tumours carry a high risk of local recurrence and distant metastases and might benefit from (neo)adjuvant treatment and more extensive surgery. Preoperative staging involves defining prognostic features of the tumour itself as well as detection of (distant) metastases (Table 1.1).

The approach of colon and rectal carcinoma involves different imaging modalities.

1.12 Staging of Colon Carcinoma

CT is recommended for staging of colon tumours. CT is used to identify patients with poor prognosis tumours based on T3 substage. These patients may benefit from neoadjuvant treatment, although up to date this is still only used in clinical trials. In regard to detection of distant metastases, CT has a high accuracy of 95%. In contrast to this, CT is not capable of identifying nodal disease. Nodal size measurements on CT have shown to be unreliable as a predictor for malignancy [7, 15, 16].

Key Points

- Colorectal cancer is the third most common cancer with more than 1,360,000 new cases diagnosed in 2012.

- The highest incidence is in North America, Australia, New Zealand and Western Europe.

- The lowest incidence is in Africa, Asia and South America.

- Anatomic site distribution: rectum 30%, colon 70%.

- Distribution within the colon: caecum 16%, ascending colon 16%, hepatic flexure 7%, transverse colon 8%, splenic flexure 5%, descending colon 6% and sigmoid 42%.

- About 30% of colorectal cancer is detected by screening of asymptomatic individuals.

- Most common chronic signs and symptoms include haematochezia or melena, abdominal pain, iron deficiency anaemia and change in bowel habit.

- There are several modalities used in screening of colorectal cancer: faecal blood testing, X-ray with barium enema, flexible sigmoidoscopy, colonoscopy and CT colonography.

- Investigation for a (suspected) colorectal cancer should be appropriately measured to the patient's comorbidities and fitness.

- Colonoscopy is regarded as the gold standard for diagnosing colorectal lesions. Colonoscopy visualises the complete colon and enables exclusion of polyps and other abnormalities.

- CT colonography has a high sensitivity of 96%, equivalent to colonoscopy for lesions ≥10 mm.

- CT colonoscopy lacks accuracy in identifying lesions smaller than 5 mm. Therefore, CT colonography is less suitable for those patients with a high risk for carcinoma or adenoma as it might miss small lesions.

- CT is recommended for staging of colon tumours. CT is used to identify patients with poor prognosis tumours based on T3 substage.

References

1. Jemal A, Bray F, Center MM, Ferlay J, Ward E, Forman D. Global cancer statistics. CA Cancer J Clin. 2011;61(2):69–90.
2. Benedix F, Kube R, Meyer F, Schmidt U, Gastinger I, Lippert H, Colon/Rectum Carcinomas (Primary Tumor) Study Group. Comparison of 17,641 patients with right- and left-sided colon cancer: differences in epidemiology, perioperative course, histology, and survival. Dis Colon Rectum. 2010;53(1):57–64.
3. Majumdar SR, Fletcher RH, Evans AT. How does colorectal cancer present? Symptoms, duration, and clues to location. Am J Gastroenterol. 1999;94(10):3039.
4. Moiel D, Thompson J. Early detection of colon cancer-the kaiser permanente northwest 30-year history: how do we measure success? Is it the test, the number of tests, the stage, or the percentage of screen-detected patients? Perm J. 2011;15(4):30–8.
5. Logan RF, Patnick J, Nickerson C, Coleman L, Rutter MD, von Wagner C, English Bowel Cancer Screening Evaluation Committee. Outcomes of the Bowel Cancer Screening Programme (BCSP) in England after the first 1 million tests. Gut. 2012;61(10):1439–46.

6. Kaminski MF, Regula J, Kraszewska E, et al. Quality indicators for colonoscopy and the risk of interval cancer. N Engl J Med. 2010;362(19):1795–803.
7. Bipat S, Glas AS, Slors FJ, Zwinderman AH, Bossuyt PM, Stoker J. Rectal cancer: local staging and assessment of lymph node involvement with endoluminal US, CT, and MR Imaging a meta-analysis. Radiology. 2004;232(3):773–83.
8. Rabeneck L, Paszat LF, Hilsden RJ, et al. Bleeding and perforation after outpatient colonoscopy and their risk factors in usual clinical practice. Astroenterology. 2008;135(6):1899–906. 1906
9. Barret M, Boustiere C, Canard JM, et al. Factors associated with adenoma detection rate and diagnosis of polyps and colorectal cancer during colonoscopy in France: results of a prospective, Nationwide survey. PLoS One. 2013;8(7):e68947.
10. Pickhardt PJ, Hassan C, Halligan S, Marmo R. Colorectal cancer: CT colonography and colonoscopy for detection systematic review and meta-analysis. Radiology. 2011;259(2): 393–405.
11. Pullens HJ, van Leeuwen MS, Laheij RJ, Vleggaar FP, Siersema PD. CT-colonography after incomplete colonoscopy: what is the diagnostic yield? Dis Colon Rectum. 2013;56(5):593–9.
12. Halligan S, Altman DG, Taylor SA, et al. CT colonography in the detection of colorectal polyps and cancer: systematic review, metaanalysis, and proposed minimum data set for study level reporting. Radiology. 2005;237(3):893–904.
13. Atkin W, Dadswell E, Wooldrage K, et al. Computed tomographic colonography versus colonoscopy for investigation of patients with symptoms suggestive of colorectal cancer (SIGGAR): a multicentre randomised trial. Lancet. 2013;381(9873):1194–202.
14. Regge D, Laudi C, Galatola G, et al. Diagnostic accuracy of computed tomographic colonography for the detection of advanced neoplasia in individuals at increased risk of colorectal cancer. JAMA. 2009;301(23):2453–61.
15. Dighe S, Blake H, Koh MD, et al. Accuracy of multidetector computed tomography in identifying poor prognostic factors in colonic cancer. Br J Surg. 2010;97(9):1407–15.
16. Dighe S, Purkayastha S, Swift I, et al. Diagnostic precision of CT in local staging of colon cancers: a meta-analysis. Clin Radiol. 2010;65(9):708–19.

Pathology of Colorectal Cancer

2

Chenggang Li

Contents

Cancer of the colon and rectum is one of the most common forms of malignancy in developed countries. It accounts for about 10% of all cancer registration in the UK, where the death rate is second only to that of lung cancer. The incidence appears to be rising. The peak incidence is between ages 60 and 79. Fewer than 20% of cases occur before age 50. Unhealthy dietary practices, obesity and physical inactivity are risk factors for colorectal cancer [1, 2].

2.1   Histological Classification of Colorectal Cancers

Roughly 25% of colorectal cancers occur in the caecum and ascending colon, 11% in the transverse colon, 6% in the descending colon and 55% in the rectosigmoid.

Histologically, these tumours are typically composed of tall columnar cells but with invasion into the submucosa, muscularis propria or beyond. A minority produce copious extracellular mucin. Carcinoma may also be poorly differentiated, solid tumours without gland formation. Less commonly, foci of neuroendocrine differentiation, signet ring cells or squamous differentiation occur. Carcinomas characteristically incite

C. Li, M.D., Ph.D., FRCPath
Warrington And Halton Hospitals NHS Foundation Trust, Warrington WA5 1QG, UK
e-mail: angiogenesisuk@yahoo.co.uk

© Springer International Publishing Switzerland 2017   9
Y. Du (ed.), *PET/CT in Colorectal Cancer*, Clinicians' Guides to Radionuclide
Hybrid Imaging - PET/CT, DOI 10.1007/978-3-319-54837-1_2

strong desmoplastic stromal responses with mesenchymal inflammation and fibrosis, leading to the firm, hard consistency of most colorectal carcinomas [3].

All colorectal carcinomas begin as in situ lesions; they evolve into different morphological patterns. Tumours in the proximal colon tend to grow as polypoid, exophytic masses that extend along one wall of the caecum and ascending colon and rarely cause obstruction. Carcinomas in the left colon tend to be annular, encircling lesions that produce constriction of the bowel. Colorectal cancers can be classified into the following histological types:

- Adenocarcinoma: this is the most common type of colorectal cancer; virtually 98% of all cancers in the large intestine are adenocarcinomas. It can be divided into three grades based on the degree of tubular or glandular formation.

Grade I accounts for 15–20% well-differentiated tumours. The majority of the tumour form well-organised tubules or glands resembling adenomatous lesion.

Grade II accounts for 60–70% moderately differentiated tumours. The amounts of tubules are between grade I and grade III tumours.

Grade III accounts for 15–20% poorly differentiated tumours. The tumours form distorted and small tubules or no tubular formation.

- Signet ring cell carcinoma: variant of adenocarcinoma with over 50% signet ring cell. This type of carcinoma is prone to metastasis and thus pursues a poor prognosis.
- Mucinous adenocarcinoma accounts for 10% of colorectal cancers and is a variant of adenocarcinoma with over 50% percent of the tumour composed of extracellular mucin.
- Small cell carcinoma accounts for less than 1% of colorectal cancers. This is a type of neuroendocrine carcinoma.
- Undifferentiated carcinoma: rare tumours, have no glandular structures or other features to indicate definite differentiation.
- Squamous and adenosquamous carcinoma: these tumours are extremely rare in the colorectum.
- Lymphomas make 1–3% of gastrointestinal malignances. Sporadic B-cell lymphomas are the most common forms. These derive from mucosa-associated lymphoid tissue (MALT).
- Carcinoid tumours: uncommon in the colorectum. Rectal carcinoids rarely metastasise, but colonic carcinoids frequently aggressive, because of their endocrine cell origin, many elaborate amines or peptides [1, 3, 5].

2.2   TNM Classification

There are two staging systems for colorectal cancer used in the UK, the TNM stage and the Dukes stage. The classification applies to carcinomas; there should be histological confirmation of the disease. The following TNM stage is based on the UICC TNM classification seventh edition [4].

Tx, primary tumour cannot be assessed

T0, no evidence of primary tumour

Tis, carcinoma in situ, intraepithelial or invasion of lamina propria

T1, tumour invades submucosa

T2, tumour invades muscularis propria

T3, tumour invades subserosa or into non-peritonised pericolic or perirectal tissues and pericolorectal tissues

T4, tumour directly invades other organs or structures and/or perforates visceral peritoneum

T4a, tumour perforates visceral peritoneum

T4b, tumour invades other organs or structures

Nx, regional lymph nodes cannot be assessed

N0, no regional lymph node metastasis

N1a, one regional lymph node

N1b, two to three regional lymph nodes

N1c, satellites without regional nodes

N2a, four to six regional nodes

N2b, seven or more regional nodes

Mx, distant metastasis cannot be assessed

M0, no distant metastasis

M1a, one organ

M1b, more than one organ, peritoneum

2.2.1 Duke Stages

Dukes A: tumour limited to muscularis propria, nodes negative

Dukes B: tumour spread beyond muscularis propria, nodes negative

Dukes C1: lymph nodes positive but highest node spared

Dukes C2: highest node involved

Dukes D: histological proven distant metastasis [3]

2.2.2 Prognostic Factors

The single most important prognostic indicator of colorectal carcinoma is the extent of the tumour at the time of diagnosis, the TNM and Dukes stage. Regardless of the system used, survival at 1, 5 and 10 years is strongly correlated with the stage of disease at the time of surgical resection. Staging can be accurately applied only after the extent of spread is determined by surgical exploration and pathological examination.

- Tumour grade: the better differentiated the tumour is, the more favourable the prognosis is. Poor differentiation predicts nodal metastatic disease.
- TNM and Dukes stage: the higher the stage, the poorer the prognosis.
- Extramural venous invasion: tumour infiltration of lymphatic or venous spaces in the submucosa or extramural spaces is regarded as a significant risk factor for lymph node or distant metastatic disease. The liver is most frequently involved.
- Lymph node metastasis: node-positive patients have significantly worse survival than those with negative nodes.

- Mismatch repair status by immunohistochemistry or microsatellite instability (MSI) testing: if abnormal, it is suggestive of unfavourable prognosis.
- K-RAS mutation: if the mutation is present, the anti-EGFR medications cetuximab (Erbitux) and panitumumab (Vectibix) are not as effective and should not be used [1, 3, 5].

Key Points

- Cancer of the colon and rectum is one of the most common forms of malignancy in developed countries.

- Roughly 25% of colorectal cancer occur in the caecum and ascending colon, 11% in the transverse colon, 6% in the descending colon and 55% in the rectosigmoid.

- Histologically, these tumours are typically composed of tall columnar cells but with invasion into the submucosa, muscularis propria or beyond.

- All colorectal carcinomas begin as in situ lesions; they evolve into different morphological patterns.

- Tumours in the proximal colon tend to grow as polypoid, exophytic masses that extend along one wall of the caecum and ascending colon and rarely cause obstruction.

- Carcinomas in the left colon tend to be annular, encircling lesions that produce constriction of the bowel. Colorectal cancers can be classified into the following histological types:

- Adenocarcinoma: this is the most common type of colorectal cancers; virtually 98% of all cancers in the large intestine are adenocarcinomas.

- The single most important prognostic indicator of colorectal carcinoma is the extent of the tumour at the time of diagnosis, the TNM and Dukes stage.

- Regardless of the system used, survival at 1, 5 and 10 years is strongly correlated with the stage of disease at the time of surgical resection.

References

1. Mills SE, editor. Sternberg's diagnostic surgical pathology. 4th ed. Baltimore: Lippincott Williams & Wilkins, 2004.
2. Fenoglio-Preiser CM, editor. Gastrointestinal pathology. 3rd ed. Baltimore: Lippincott Williams & Wilkins, 2008.
3. Fletcher CDM, editor. Diagnostic histopathology. 3rd ed. USA: Churchill Livingstone Elsevier, 2007.
4. Sobin L, et al., editors. TNM classification of malignant tumour, UICC international union against cancer. 7th ed. UK: Wiley-Blackwell, 2009.
5. Mitchell R, et al., editors. Robbins and Cotran Pathologic basis of disease. 7th ed. Philadelphia: Saunders Elsevier 2006.

Management of Colorectal Cancer

3

Gayathri Anandappa

Contents

Over recent decades there has been a marked improvement in survival outcomes of patients with CRC. A number of factors have contributed to this including earlier diagnosis through the utilisations of two-week rule referral pathways, the adoption of an MDT approach to management, refinements to the surgical management,

G. Anandappa
The Royal Marsden Hospital NHS Foundation Trust,
203 Fulham Rd, Chelsea, London SW3 6JJ, UK
e-mail: Gayathri.Anandappa@rmh.nhs.uk

© Springer International Publishing Switzerland 2017
Y. Du (ed.), *PET/CT in Colorectal Cancer*, Clinicians' Guides to Radionuclide
Hybrid Imaging - PET/CT, DOI 10.1007/978-3-319-54837-1_3

13

improved staging including the utilising of MRI and PET in selected cases, developments in systemic chemotherapy and improved follow-up assessments.

3.1   Role of the Multidisciplinary Team (MDT)

The treatment plan for any individual patient is indicated by a number of factors, including:

- Primary site of disease (colon vs rectum)
- Stage of the tumour
- Patient factors including co-morbidities and performance status.

Localised colonic tumours are frequently managed with primary surgery. For rectal tumours neoadjuvant strategies utilising radiotherapy or chemoradiotherapy may be utilised to minimise the risk of subsequent local disease recurrence. A proportion of patients will present with oligometastatic disease (most commonly liver metastasis) that may be amenable to a curative approach. The multidisciplinary team input is key to achieving the optimal patient outcomes.

3.2   Management of Localised Disease

3.2.1   Surgery for Localised Disease

- Early T1 tumours: A small proportion of patients with early T1 tumours (with limited submucosal involvement) considered at low risk of nodal involvement may be amenable to removal by endoscopic mucosal resection.
- Localised colonic tumours are treated as follows:
    - Right hemicolectomy is performed for tumours of caecum, ascending colon and proximal transverse colon.
    - Tumours of descending and upper sigmoid colon are removed by left hemicolectomy.
    - Distal sigmoid and upper and mid rectal tumours are removed by anterior resection.
- It has been shown that there is no difference between open and laparoscopic approaches in experienced hands.
- It is important to achieve reasonable nodal clearance and a minimum of 8 and ideally at least >12 nodes is recommended for adequate staging. If lymph node clearance is not adequate, then there is a risk of under-staging.
- In patients presenting with complications, i.e. obstruction or perforation, emergency decompression and resection, can be performed as a one-stage or two-stage procedure with a stoma. Emergency surgery is associated with higher perioperative mortality due to poor nutritional status of patients, poor bowel preparation and locally advanced disease and higher rates of recurrence.

3.2.2   Rectal Tumours

- There have been significant improvements in local control rates with the adoption of total mesorectal excision (TME) surgery and the use of pre-op chemoradiotherapy or radiotherapy.
- In patients with rectal tumours, pelvic MRI is used to stage the local disease and nodes and relationship of tumour with mesorectal fascia. A distance of <2 mm between the primary tumour and the mesorectal fascia is predictive of potential involvement of circumferential resection margin (CRM) (<1 mm) following surgery. With the development of TME for rectal tumours, local recurrence rates have reduced from >20% to <10% [1, 2].
- Lower rectal tumours can be excised by abdomino-perineal resection with removal of the anal canal and a permanent stoma; more recently, however, there has been a shift towards low anastomosis without stoma.

3.3   Adjuvant Treatment in Localised Disease

3.3.1   Chemotherapy

- Adjuvant chemotherapy for 6 months with 5-fluorouracil or capecitabine with or without oxaliplatin has demonstrated benefit for patients with stage III disease [3, 4] (please see metastatic section for more details on chemotherapy).
- In patients with stage II disease, the benefit is more modest and adjuvant chemotherapy with single agent capecitabine is recommended in patients with the following high risk factors:
  - T4 tumours
  - Number of nodes examined not adequate
  - Poorly or undifferentiated tumours
  - Emergency presentation
  - Presence of extramural vascular invasion
- In patients with stage II disease with microsatellite instability (MSI), adjuvant chemotherapy is not recommended.

3.4   Radiotherapy

- Radiotherapy has an important role in patients with rectal tumours in the neoadjuvant and adjuvant setting, to either downsize locally advanced rectal tumours to render them resectable or to prevent local recurrence [5].
- Both short-course (25Gy in 5 fractions) and conventionally fractionated (45–50.4Gy in 1.8–2.0Gy/fraction) preoperative radiotherapy have demonstrated improved local control [6, 7]. Chemoradiotherapy has shown to be more effective than radiotherapy alone in resectable disease. In locally advanced rectal tumours, neoadjuvant concurrent chemoradiotherapy is the standard of care [8–10].

3.4.1 Follow-Up

Following adjuvant treatment patients are followed up every 3 months with tumour marker CEA (carcinoembryonic antigen) and annual CT scans up to 3 years to identify any early relapses especially oligo-metastatic disease which may be amenable to curative surgery.

3.5 Treatment of Metastatic Colorectal Cancer (mCRC)

- Around 30% of patients with mCRC present with stage IV or advanced disease and ~25% of patients treated with localised disease develop recurrent disease. PET/CT plays a key role in the delineation of the metastatic burden.
- Historically, median overall survival with best supportive care is less than 6 months.
- Treatment with systemic chemotherapy increases overall survival up to 20 months.
- Patients with metastatic disease need to undergo testing of the *RAS/RAF* status. Patients with mutations in *RAS/RAF* pathway do not respond to epidermal growth factor (EGFR)-targeted therapy. Recent data suggest that in patients with wild-type *RAS/RAF*, overall survival of up to 30 months can be achieved with the use of targeted agents. *BRAF* mutations are associated with poor prognosis and seen in 5–11% of patients with mCRC [11, 12].
- Surgery is used in the advanced setting for potentially resectable disease in the liver or lungs or for palliation of symptoms.

3.6 Systemic Therapy

3.6.1 Cytotoxics

3.6.1.1 Fluropyrimidine-Based Therapy
- 5-FU is the backbone of the chemotherapeutic regimens used in advanced disease in first- and second-line settings. It works by inhibition of thymidylate synthase (TS), thereby inhibiting DNA synthesis. It is co-administered with folinic acid, which stabilises the interaction with TS. It can be administered as an infusion or bolus, with infusion having less marrow suppression.
- Capecitabine, an oral prodrug of 5-FU, has equal efficacy to 5-FU [13]. In meta-analyses, 5-FU-based regimens prolong median survival by 12 months. Side effects of infusional 5-FU include diarrhoea; capecitabine has comparatively much higher incidence of diarrhoea, mucositis and hand-foot syndrome. Coronary vasospasm is another side effect that limits use of 5-FU/capecitabine and raltitrexed is used in such patients.

3.6.1.2 Doublet-Chemotherapy Regimens
5-FU or capecitabine is combined with oxaliplatin or irinotecan.

- Oxaliplatin is platinum-based chemotherapy that binds with DNA, forming intra- and interstrand adducts, which are cleared by DNA damage pathways. The main side effect with oxaliplatin is cumulative sensory neuropathy and is a dose-limiting toxicity. Combination of 5-FU with oxaliplatin (FOLFOX) improves progression-free survival but not overall survival; combining oxaliplatin with capecitabine showed equal efficacy and tolerability [13].
- Irinotecan causes DNA single-strand breaks by inhibiting topoisomerase 1 leading to apoptosis. Severe diarrhoea is a well-recognised side effect of irinotecan, and early initiation of anti-diarrhoeal therapy is recommended. Irinotecan in combination with infusional 5-FU (FOLFIRI) was reasonably well tolerated and improved response rates and overall survival in phase III trials [14]. Combining irinotecan with capecitabine, however, led to excessive diarrhoea and is not commonly used.

3.7 Targeted Agents

3.7.1 Bevacizumab

- Bevacizumab, a humanised monoclonal antibody against VEGF ligand, is an anti-angiogenic agent used in the first-line setting in combination with 5-FU/capecitabine and oxaliplatin [15].
- Hypertension and proteinuria are common side effects with the drug. Arterial thromboembolic events [16], haemorrhage, perforation and fistula formation are much rarer but serious side effects with bevacizumab. The risk of perforation is increased with recent surgery and peritoneal disease.

3.8 Cetuximab

- In patients with wild-type K-Ras, cetuximab, an anti-EGFR chimeric antibody, offers a small survival benefit over best supportive care in the third-line setting.
- In a select group of patients, it can be used in combination with chemotherapy in the first-line setting [17].
- An acneiform rash is a common side effect with cetuximab, and treatment with tetracycline-based antibiotics is now part of prophylaxis.

3.9 Aflibercept

Aflibercept, a VEGF trap antibody, has shown improved overall survival when used in combination with FOLFIRI in patients with mCRC after treatment with an oxaliplatin-based regimen, including bevacizumab-treated patients [18].

3.10 Regorafenib

Regorafenib is a small molecule multi-kinase inhibitor that has shown overall survival benefit in patients with mCRC who have progressed after standard lines of treatment [19].

3.11 Role of Surgery in Advanced Colorectal Cancer

- Metastatic disease is most commonly limited to the liver with a small percentage of patients presenting with lung metastases.
- Resection of liver-only metastases results in a 30% improved 5-year survival in patients with advanced disease. 10% of patients have liver metastases that is resectable at presentation and 10% of patients have metastases that can be downstaged by chemotherapy and then resected.
- In symptomatic patients with obstruction or bleeding, palliative surgery is performed as a semi-elective procedure or as an emergency. The use of colonic or rectal stents to relieve obstruction remains controversial and has been associated with high rates of perforation in few studies.

3.12 Other Modalities of Treatment

Radiofrequency ablation has a role in the treatment of liver metastases and lung metastases. Patients need to be selected carefully in a MDT setting for these treatments.

Conclusion

Patients with colorectal cancer have numerous treatment options, and personalising treatment care in a MDT setting achieves better survival outcomes. PET imaging plays an important role in the diagnostic pathway and management of these patients.

Key Points

- The treatment plan for any individual patient is indicated by a number of factors, including primary site of disease (colon vs rectum), stage of the tumour, patient factors including co-morbidities and performance status.

- Localised colonic tumours are frequently managed with primary surgery.

- Right hemicolectomy (tumours of caecum, ascending colon and proximal transverse colon).

- Left hemicolectomy (tumours of descending and upper sigmoid colon)

- Anterior resection (distal sigmoid and upper and mid rectal tumours)

- In patients with rectal tumours, neoadjuvant strategies utilising radiotherapy or chemoradiotherapy may be utilised to minimise the risk of subsequent local disease recurrence.

- Lower rectal tumours can be excised by abdomino-perineal resection with removal of the anal canal and a permanent stoma; more recently, however, there has been a shift towards low anastomosis without stoma:

  - Adjuvant chemotherapy for 6 months with 5-fluorouracil or capecitabine with or without oxaliplatin has demonstrated benefit for patients with stage III disease.

  - Radiotherapy has an important role in patients with rectal tumours in the neoadjuvant and adjuvant setting, to either downsize locally advanced rectal tumours to render them resectable or to prevent local recurrence.

- Around 30% of patients with mCRC present with stage IV or advanced disease, and ~25% of patients treated with localised disease develop recurrent disease. PET/CT plays a key role in the delineation of the metastatic burden.

- Metastatic disease is most commonly limited to the liver with a small percentage of patients presenting with lung metastases.

- Resection of liver-only metastases results in a 30% improved 5-year survival in patients with advanced disease.

- Radiofrequency ablation has a role in the treatment of liver metastases and lung metastases.

References

1. Heald RJ, Ryall RD. Recurrence and survival after total mesorectal excision for rectal cancer. Lancet. 1986;1(8496):1479–82.
2. Peeters KC, Marijnen CA, Nagtegaal ID, et al. The TME trial after a median follow-up of 6 years: increased local control but no survival benefit in irradiated patients with resectable rectal carcinoma. Ann Surg. 2007;246(5):693–701.
3. Andre T, Boni C, Mounedji-Boudiaf L, et al. Oxaliplatin, fluorouracil, and leucovorin as adjuvant treatment for colon cancer. N Engl J Med. 2004;350(23):2343–51.
4. Kuebler JP, Wieand HS, O'Connell MJ, et al. Oxaliplatin combined with weekly bolus fluorouracil and leucovorin as surgical adjuvant chemotherapy for stage II and III colon cancer: results from NSABP C-07. J Clin Oncol Off J Am Soc Clin Oncol. 2007;25(16):2198–204.
5. Camma C, Giunta M, Fiorica F, Pagliaro L, Craxi A, Cottone M. Preoperative radiotherapy for resectable rectal cancer: a meta-analysis. JAMA. 2000;284(8):1008–15.

6. Bujko K, Nowacki MP, Nasierowska-Guttmejer A, Michalski W, Bebenek M, Kryj M. Long-term results of a randomized trial comparing preoperative short-course radiotherapy with preoperative conventionally fractionated chemoradiation for rectal cancer. Br J Surg. 2006;93(10):1215–23.

7. Bosset JF, Collette L, Calais G, et al. Chemotherapy with preoperative radiotherapy in rectal cancer. N Engl J Med. 2006;355(11):1114–23.

8. Gerard JP, Conroy T, Bonnetain F, et al. Preoperative radiotherapy with or without concurrent fluorouracil and leucovorin in T3-4 rectal cancers: results of FFCD 9203. J Clin Oncol Off J Am Soc Clin Oncol. 2006;24(28):4620–5.

9. Kapiteijn E, Marijnen CA, Nagtegaal ID, et al. Preoperative radiotherapy combined with total mesorectal excision for resectable rectal cancer. N Engl J Med. 2001;345(9):638–46.

10. Sebag-Montefiore D, Stephens RJ, Steele R, et al. Preoperative radiotherapy versus selective postoperative chemoradiotherapy in patients with rectal cancer (MRC CR07 and NCIC-CTG C016): a multicentre, randomised trial. Lancet. 2009;373(9666):811–20.

11. Tran B, Kopetz S, Tie J, et al. Impact of BRAF mutation and microsatellite instability on the pattern of metastatic spread and prognosis in metastatic colorectal cancer. Cancer. 2011;117(20):4623–32.

12. Yokota T, Ura T, Shibata N, et al. BRAF mutation is a powerful prognostic factor in advanced and recurrent colorectal cancer. Br J Cancer. 2011;104(5):856–62.

13. Rothenberg ML, Cox JV, Butts C, et al. Capecitabine plus oxaliplatin (XELOX) versus 5-fluorouracil/folinic acid plus oxaliplatin (FOLFOX-4) as second-line therapy in metastatic colorectal cancer: a randomized phase III noninferiority study. Ann Oncol. 2008;19(10):1720–6.

14. Douillard JY, Cunningham D, Roth AD, et al. Irinotecan combined with fluorouracil compared with fluorouracil alone as first-line treatment for metastatic colorectal cancer: a multicentre randomised trial. Lancet. 2000;355(9209):1041–7.

15. Hurwitz HI, Fehrenbacher L, Hainsworth JD, et al. Bevacizumab in combination with fluorouracil and leucovorin: an active regimen for first-line metastatic colorectal cancer. J Clin Oncol Off J Am Soc Clin Oncol. 2005;23(15):3502–8.

16. Scappaticci FA, Skillings JR, Holden SN, et al. Arterial thromboembolic events in patients with metastatic carcinoma treated with chemotherapy and bevacizumab. J Natl Cancer Inst. 2007;99(16):1232–9.

17. Heinemann V, von Weikersthal LF, Decker T, et al. FOLFIRI plus cetuximab versus FOLFIRI plus bevacizumab as first-line treatment for patients with metastatic colorectal cancer (FIRE-3): a randomised, open-label, phase 3 trial. Lancet Oncol. 2014;15(10):1065–75.

18. Van Cutsem E, Tabernero J, Lakomy R, et al. Addition of aflibercept to fluorouracil, leucovorin, and irinotecan improves survival in a phase III randomized trial in patients with metastatic colorectal cancer previously treated with an oxaliplatin-based regimen. J Clin Oncol Off J Am Soc Clin Oncol. 2012;30(28):3499–506.

19. Grothey A, Van Cutsem E, Sobrero A, et al. Regorafenib monotherapy for previously treated metastatic colorectal cancer (CORRECT): an international, multicentre, randomised, placebo-controlled, phase 3 trial. Lancet. 2013;381(9863):303–12.

Radiological Imaging of Colorectal Cancer

4

Svetlana Balyasnikova and Gina Brown

Contents

Colon cancers are staged using CT as follows: oral administration of 1 l water to delineate the small and large bowel and 100–150 ml intravenous iodinated contrast medium injected at 3–4 ml/s. Multidetector CT scans are acquired at 20–25 s (chest) and 70–80 s (abdomen and pelvis) post-injection with sections acquired at 1.25–2.5 mm section thickness and reformatted in the axial, sagittal and coronal planes at 2–5 mm for viewing. The image analysis is performed on a workstation with three-dimensional reconstruction software. This enables the images to be viewed in the coronal and sagittal planes and also allows rotation of the images for optimum comprehensive analysis.

4.1 Staging of Colon Cancers Using CT

A meta-analysis showed that the sensitivity and specificity of differentiating between T1/T2 vs. T3/T4 was 86% and 78%, respectively, using multidetector CT techniques, the pooled sensitivity and specificity for detecting tumour invasion in studies was 93% and 86%, respectively [1].

S. Balyasnikova (✉) • G. Brown
Department of Radiology, The Royal Marsden NHS Foundation Trust, London, UK
e-mail: Svetlana.Balyasnikova@rmh.nhs.uk

© Springer International Publishing Switzerland 2017
Y. Du (ed.), *PET/CT in Colorectal Cancer*, Clinicians' Guides to Radionuclide Hybrid Imaging - PET/CT, DOI 10.1007/978-3-319-54837-1_4

- Tumours are only classified as having poor prognosis if tumour extension is 5 mm beyond the muscularis propria. For colon cancers applying the TNM classification system, tumours are grouped on the following basis: good prognosis tumours are T1/T2, T3a and T3b (>80% 3 year DFS), whereas poor prognosis tumours are T3c, T3d and T4 and have significantly poorer DFS [2].
- **T1, T2 and early T3 tumours.** According to the TNM staging system, T1 and T2 tumours are defined as follows: T1, tumour limited to the mucosa; T2, tumour extending to the submucosa, but not involving the muscularis propria. On CT scans, T1 tumours produce an intraluminal projection or focal mass without any visible distortion of the bowel wall layers. T2 tumours are tumours with greater asymmetrical thickening projecting intraluminally but with preservation of smooth muscle coat.

Tumours can be best confirmed as early stage on the multiplanar reformatted sections, where the lack of infiltration through the bowel wall can be appreciated.

- **T3 tumours** are those that infiltrate beyond the muscularis propria. The features on CT suggestive of poor prognosis T3 infiltration (T3c and T3d) include smooth or nodular extension of a discrete mass of tumour tissue beyond the contour of the bowel wall with extension into pericolic fat >5 mm [3].
- **Retroperitoneal fascia invasion.** Further high-risk features include infiltration of the retroperitoneal fascia; this is the posterior surgical resection margin for the tumours lying in the ascending and descending colon, and unless colonic dissection is extended, such patients are at risk of incomplete resection.
- **T4 tumours.** CT features to identify a T4 tumour include the presence of nodular penetration of the tumour through the peritonealised areas of the muscle coat or an advancing edge of the tumour penetrating adjacent organs. Peritoneal infiltration is an independent prognostic factor, and its presence worsens the patient's prognosis [4–5].
- **Nodal stage.** The accurate detection of nodal status has always been difficult using CT. The limitation of CT to detect micro-metastasis in the nodes leads to poor accuracy. The sensitivities and specificities for detection of nodal status range from 66 to 83% and 35 to 81%, respectively. It is not recommended that CT is used to assess the likelihood of nodal malignancy due to substantial overlap between benign enlarged inflammatory nodes and malignant nodes.
- Extramural venous invasion is an independent prognostic factor in colorectal cancers. EMVI can be seen using CT as definite enhancing tumour spread along a large vein, e.g. the ileocolic vein, superior rectal vein, etc [6].

4.2   Assessment of Rectal Cancers

Imaging is essential for both primary and recurrent rectal cancer, for baseline staging and tumour response assessment. MRI has become the optimal modality for the local staging of primary tumours. There are several advantages over alternative techniques; it enables risk stratification of tumours depending on the presence of high-risk features and characteristics (T and N stages, CRM and EMVI status) that are proven to influence disease-free and overall survival rates [7–9]. In recurrent rectal cancer, MRI enables delineation of tumour extent within the pelvic compartments, assesses the pattern of local recurrence and predicts resectability of the tumour. According to global standards, patients with locally advanced tumours should receive preoperative therapy (usually, radiotherapy in combination with chemotherapy). MRI has also been shown to be a reliable tool in assessment of tumour response to preoperative treatment [10].

4.3   Summary of Rectal MRI Assessment Standards for Reporting

4.3.1   Baseline and Post-treatment Assessment of Rectal Cancer MRI

Confirm high-resolution scan using correct parameters (in plane resolution 0.6×0.6 mm, voxel size 1.1 mm^3), correct scan planes orthogonal to long axis of tumour and adequate coverage that includes the mesorectum up to L5/S1.

4.3.2   Minimum Standards for Reporting:

1. **Description of primary tumour morphology:**
   - **Morphologic types:** annular/semi-annular/ulcerating/polypoidal/mucinous mass
   - **Description of the invasive border** of the tumour: nodular infiltrating vs. smooth "pushing" border
2. **Assessment of height:**
   - **Height from anal verge** (defined as lower border of internal sphincter fibres)
   - **Assessment of height of tumour above the sphincter complex** (defined as the upper border of puborectalis sling)
   - **Relationship of tumour to the anterior peritoneal reflection** (below/at/ above)
   - **Quadrant** and extent of the invading border
3. **Depth of spread** beyond the muscularis propria of tumour spread (millimetres).
4. **T substage:** T1 (sm1/sm2/sm3); T2 inner fibres/full thickness; T3a (<1 mm spread), T3b (1–5 mm), T3c (5–15 mm) and T3d >15 mm; T4 visceral invasion or T4 peritoneal infiltration.
5. **Relationship of tumour to the intersphincteric plane for tumours arising 6 cm or less from the anal verge.**

- Tumour confined to the submucosal layer or only part thickness of muscularis propria indicates that the intersphincteric plane/mesorectal plane is safe and intersphincteric APE or ultralow TME would be possible.
- Tumour extending through the full thickness of the muscularis propria at or below the puborectalis sling indicates that intersphincteric plane/mesorectal plane is unsafe; in such patients, extralevator APE is required for radial clearance.
- Tumour extending into the intersphincteric plane means that the intersphincteric plane/mesorectal plane is unsafe; therefore, an extralevator APE is also indicated for radial clearance.
- Tumour extends into the external sphincter: intersphincteric plane/mesorectal plane is unsafe, and extralevator APE is indicated for radial clearance.
- Tumour extending into adjacent prostate/vagina/bladder/sacrum indicates that an exenterative procedure would be required.

6. **Lymph node** assessment should not be based on the diameter of the node but instead based on assessment of heterogeneity or irregularity of border to assess risk of malignancy. Smooth-bordered and uniform signal nodes are defined as benign based on MRI criteria.

7. **Extramural venous invasion:** tumour extension into veins either contiguous with the main tumour or discontinuous—characterised by irregular expansion of the calibre of the vessel by tumour signal.

8. **CRM is assessed** by measuring the closest distance of tumour to the mesorectal fascia by tumour in millimetres and stating the location of the potential margin and the cause (tumour, vascular invasion or tumour deposit). The potential CRM is defined as involved if the measured distance to the mesorectal fascia is 1 mm or less. A distance >1 mm indicates that the potential CRM is clear.

9. **Peritoneal dissemination:** an assessment of the pelvic cavity is undertaken to search for potential peritoneal deposits; this is particularly important for anterior tumours that have infiltrated beyond the peritoneal membrane.

10. **Pelvic side wall lymph nodes** can be assessed by evaluating the common sites of lateral spread, i.e. the obturator fossa, external iliac nodes and internal iliac nodes. Assessment should not be based on the diameter of the node but instead based on assessment of heterogeneity or irregularity of border to assess risk of malignancy. Smooth-bordered and uniform signal nodes are defined as benign based on MRI criteria.

Summary of stage should be given—this should include mrT substage, mrN status, CRM EMVI and assessment of the pelvic side wall nodes.

Tumours with <5 mm extramural spread, safe CRM and absence of EMVI do not present a risk of local recurrence and are thus eligible for primary surgery.

Poor prognosis tumours (T3c or greater, EMVI positive or CRM positive) are eligible for preoperative chemoradiotherapy.

Following treatment, the same assessment is undertaken measuring areas of residual tumour signal and the same definitions as pretreatment scans. In addition, an mrTRG assessment is undertaken:

- If the treated tumour shows no fibrosis, this is classified as mrTRG5.
- If the treated tumour shows minimal fibrosis and predominant tumour signal, this is defined as mrTRG4.
- If there is predominant fibrosis but macroscopic tumour remains, mrTRG 3.
- If there is fibrosis, with minimal or no tumour signal intensity, mrTRG2 (near-complete response).
- If there is low signal fibrosis, linear scar only and no intermediate tumour signal, this is mrTRG1 (radiologic complete response)

Key Points

- The sensitivity and specificity of differentiating between T1/T2 and T3/T4 was 86% and 78%, respectively, using multidetector CT techniques.

- The pooled sensitivity and specificity of CT for detecting tumour invasion in studies is 93% and 86%, respectively.

- Tumours are only classified as having poor prognosis if tumour extension is 5 mm beyond the muscularis propria.

- Colon cancers with good prognosis are T1/T2, T3a and T3b tumours (>80% 3-year DFS).

- Colon cancers with poor prognosis are T3c, T3d and T4 tumours and have significantly poorer DFS.

- The accurate detection of nodal status has always been difficult using CT. The limitation of CT to detect micro-metastasis in the nodes leads to poor accuracy.

- Sensitivities and specificities for detection of nodal status range from 66 to 83% and 35 to 81%, respectively.

- It is not recommended that CT is used to assess the likelihood of nodal malignancy due to substantial overlap between benign enlarged inflammatory nodes and malignant nodes.

- Extramural venous invasion is an independent prognostic factor in colorectal cancers.

- Imaging is essential for both primary and recurrent rectal cancer, for baseline staging and tumour response assessment. MRI has become the optimal modality for the local staging of primary tumours.

References

1. Dighe S, Purkayastha S, Swift I, Tekkis PP, Darzi A, A'Hern R, Brown G. Diagnostic precision of CT in local staging of colon cancers: a meta-analysis. Clin Radiol. 2010;65(9):708–19.
2. Smith NJ, Bees N, Barbachano Y, et al. Preoperative computed tomography staging of non-metastatic colon cancer predicts outcome: implications for clinical trials. Br J Cancer. 2007;96:1030–6.
3. Burton S, Brown G, Bees N, et al. Accuracy of CT prediction of poor prognostic features in colonic cancer. Br J Radiol. 2008;81:10–9.
4. Shepherd NA, Baxter KJ, Love SB. The prognostic importance of peritoneal involvement in colonic cancer: a prospective evaluation. Gastroenterology. 1997;112:1096–102.
5. Lennon AM, Mulcahy HE, Hyland JMP, et al. Peritoneal involvement in stage II colon cancer. Am J Clin Pathol. 2003;119:108–13.
6. Dighe S, Blake H, Koh MD, Swift I, Arnaout A, Temple L, Barbachano Y, Brown G. Accuracy of multidetector computed tomography in identifying poor prognostic factors in colonic cancer. Br J Surg. 2010;97(9):1407–15. doi:10.1002/bjs.7096.
7. Brown G, et al. Preoperative assessment of prognostic factors in rectal cancer using high-resolution magnetic resonance imaging. Br J Surg. 2003;90(3):355–64.
8. Taylor FG, et al. Preoperative magnetic resonance imaging assessment of circumferential resection margin predicts disease-free survival and local recurrence: 5- year follow-up results of the MERCURY study. J Clin Oncol. 2014;32(1):34–43.
9. Smith NJ, et al. Prognostic significance of magnetic resonance imaging-detected extramural vascular invasion in rectal cancer. Br J Surg. 2008;95(2):229–36.
10. Patel UB, et al. Magnetic resonance imaging-detected tumor response for locally advanced rectal cancer predicts survival outcomes: MERCURY experience. J Clin Oncol. 2011; 29(28):3753–60.

¹⁸F-FDG PET/CT: Normal Variants, Artefacts, and Pitfalls in Colorectal Cancer

5

Arun Sasikumar and Ajith Joy

Contents

A. Sasikumar (✉) • A. Joy
Department of Nuclear Medicine and PET/CT, KIMS-DDNMRC, Trivandrum, India
e-mail: drarunddnmrc@gmail.com; sasikumararun@gmail.com

© Springer International Publishing Switzerland 2017
Y. Du (ed.), *PET/CT in Colorectal Cancer*, Clinicians' Guides to Radionuclide
Hybrid Imaging - PET/CT, DOI 10.1007/978-3-319-54837-1_5

5.1   Introduction

Colorectal cancer is the third most common cancer worldwide and the second most common cancer in Europe. The role of ^{18}F-FDG (FDG) PET/CT in suspected recurrence, in patients with liver metastases eligible for surgical management, and in treatment response evaluation in colorectal carcinoma is now well established with more data emerging in initial staging of colorectal cancer [1]. FDG PET/CT can influence the management strategies in colorectal patient in up to 30% of the cases [2]. In this context, adequate understanding of the physiological variants, possible artefacts, as well as imaging pitfalls of FDG PET/CT in colorectal carcinoma patients is extremely important.

5.2   Physiological Variants

A thorough understanding of sites of physiological uptake in abdomen and pelvis (Fig. 5.1) is an essential prerequisite to interpret FDG PET/CT scans in colorectal carcinoma. Physiologically increased FDG uptake is seen in the diaphragmatic cruces in conditions of increased abdominal breathing effort (Fig. 5.2). Perhaps FDG uptake in the gastrointestinal tract is the most variable (Fig. 5.3) ranging from no

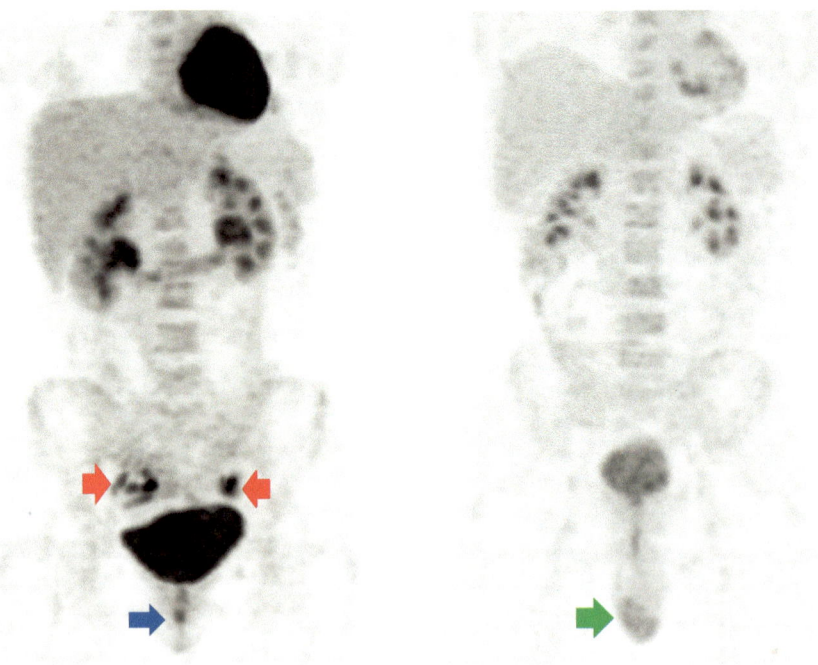

Fig. 5.1 Physiological FDG uptake in the abdomen and pelvis: Usually most intense FDG activity is noted in the pelvicalyceal system, ureters, and urinary bladder. Physiological but less intense FDG uptake is noted in the liver, spleen, bone marrow, and renal cortices. Physiological (variable) FDG uptake may be seen in the uterus and ovaries (*red arrows*) depending on the phase of menstrual cycle. Physiological (low to moderate grade) FDG uptake may be seen in the testes (*green arrow*). Focal FDG uptake at the anus (*blue arrow*) is due to sphincter activation or local inflammation

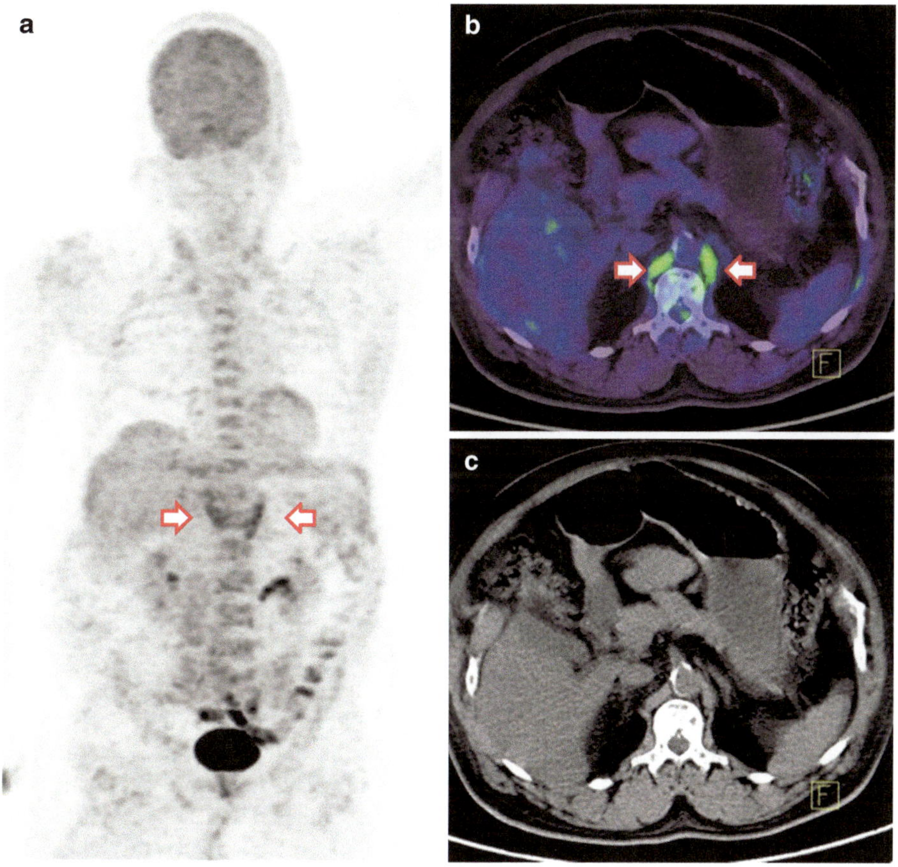

Fig. 5.2 FDG uptake in bilateral diaphragmatic cruses (**a - MIP**). Physiological nature of the uptake can be ascertained by the symmetrical nature of FDG uptake (**b**) and absence of any lesion in the CT part (**c**)

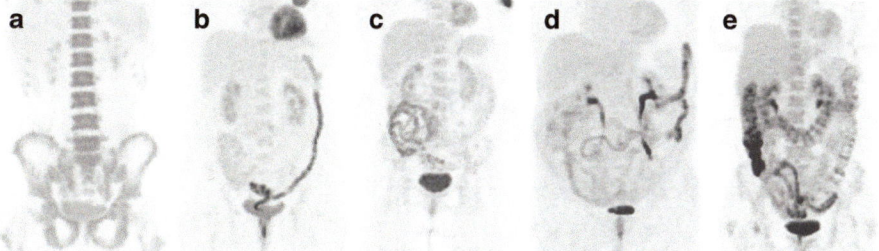

Fig. 5.3 Physiological uptake pattern in large and small bowel. It can range from absent uptake (**a**) to segmental (**b, c**), patchy (**d**), or diffuse uptake (**e**)

discernible uptake above background to diffuse intense FDG uptake [3] and may be affected by a number of factors ranging from smooth muscle contraction to mucosal metabolic activity [4].

5.3 Artefacts and Imaging Pitfalls

Potential artefacts and imaging pitfalls in the interpretation of FDG PET/CT in colorectal cancers are mostly related to abdomen and pelvic regions. They can be broadly grouped into technical: organ or pathology specific and treatment related.

5.4 Technical Artefacts

5.4.1 Misregistration

Misregistration is an incorrect superimposition of PET and CT data on a fused image, potentially resulting in an abnormality being ascribed to the wrong structure. It may be due to breathing, patient motion, bowel motility, or distension of the bladder and can result in both false-positive or false-negative PET findings if not identified and corrected appropriately [5]. Respiratory motion artefacts (Fig. 5.4) predominantly affect structures close to the diaphragm especially liver lesions and basal lung lesions. Review of PET alone images and identification of any associated CT abnormalities would be helpful. Patient motion and consequent artefacts are minimised by (a) placing the patient in a comfortable position, (b) instructing patient not to move during the study, and (c) having the patients empty their bladder before the start of the study. Acquisition of PET images from pelvis to head, after CT acquisition, also helps in reducing artefacts due to bladder filling (Fig. 5.5). Bowel peristalsis and positional changes also result in misregistration (Fig. 5.6),

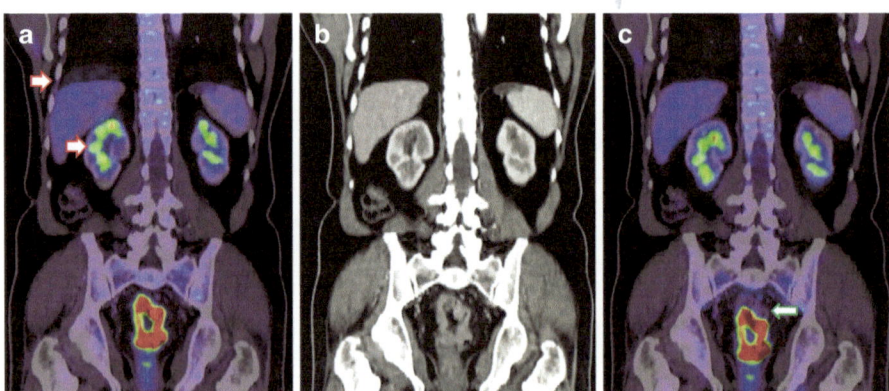

Fig. 5.4 Misregistration of liver and renal FDG uptake (**a - coronal fused PET/CT, b - corornal contrast enhanced CT**) due to respiratory movement (*red arrows*). (**c**) Images after manual correction for misregistration of liver and renal activity, but it induces misregistration at the site of pathological FDG uptake in the lesion in the rectum (*green arrow*). Care should be taken while interpreting images with misregistration

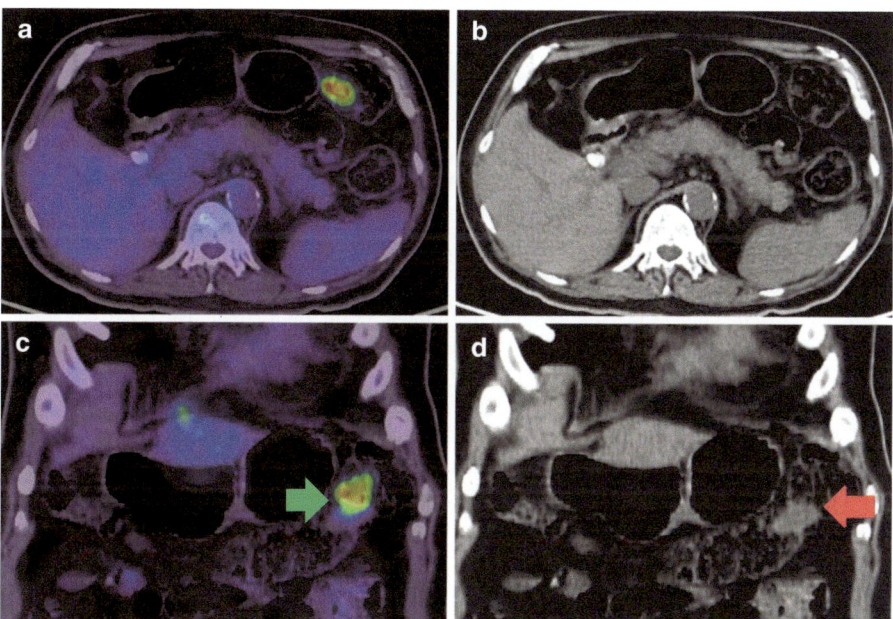

Fig. 5.5 Misregistration due to bowel movement. Intensely FDG concentration in the left third of the transverse colon (**a**) with no corresponding lesion seen in CT (**b**). Careful review of coronal images (**c - coronal fused PET/CT and d - coronal CT images**) reveals the misregistration (*green arrow*—FDG uptake and *red arrow*, lesion in CT)

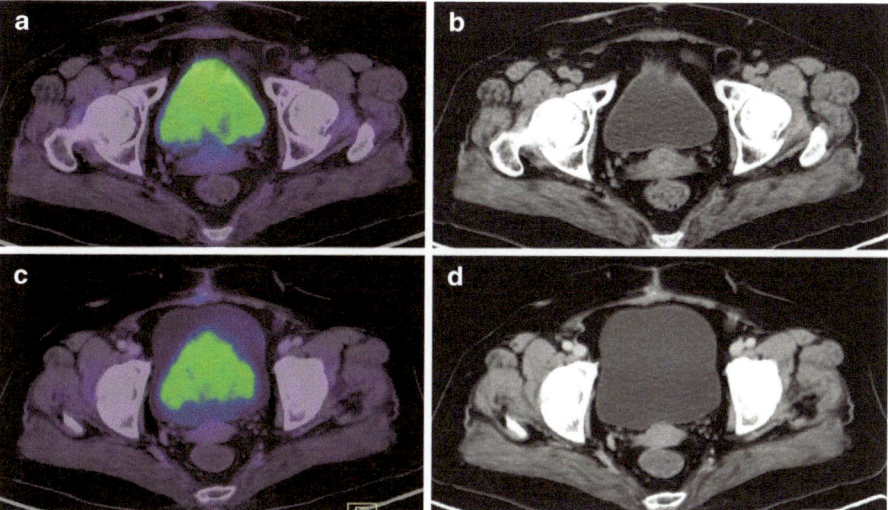

Fig. 5.6 Bladder misregistration—fused PET/CT (**a**) images and corresponding section of plain CT (**b**) used for fusion. Contrast-enhanced CT was acquired after plain CT without changing the patient position. Misregistered PET/CECT image (**c**) and corresponding section of contrastenhanced CT (**d**) used for fusion

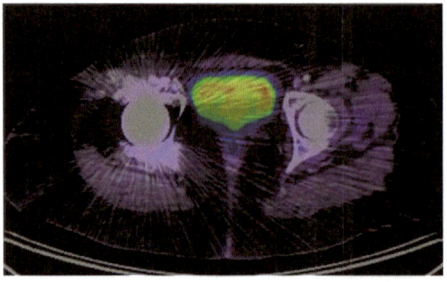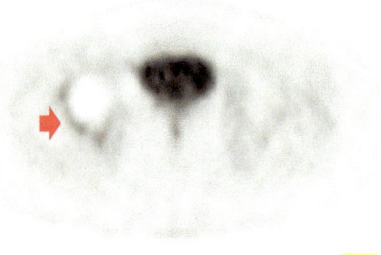

Fig. 5.7 Artefact due to metallic orthopaedic implant in the right femur. The CT-based attenuation map corrects (or overcorrects) photopenic areas adjacent to high-attenuation structures and makes them appear hypermetabolic on the attenuation-corrected PET images (*red arrow*). Review of PET images alone and attenuation noncorrected images would be helpful

particularly in the small bowel. Potential use of antiperistaltic agents like *N*-butylscopolamine exists but requires further studies and validation [6].

5.4.2   Partial Volume Effect

In PET scanners, spatial resolution effects can lead to underestimation of activity in small lesions with consequent pitfalls in assessing small moderately active lesions, where modest changes in apparent activity may influence interpretation [7].

5.4.3   Attenuation Correction Artefacts

It is seen in the presence of highly attenuating objects like metallic prostheses/stents, high-density drainage tubes, and dense intravenous contrast in the path of the CT beam (Fig. 5.7). These artefacts can easily be identified by comparing the attenuation-corrected images with the uncorrected images. [8].

5.4.4   Truncation Artefacts

Truncation artefacts in PET/CT are essentially due to the difference in size of the axial field of view between the CT (50 cm) and the PET (70 cm) tomographs. Modern scanners mitigate these effects by reconstructing attenuation correction maps to 70 cm using data extrapolation methods [9, 10].

5.5   Organ- and Pathology-Specific Pitfalls

5.5.1   Liver

Physiological FDG uptake is homogeneous/uniformly mottled and slightly greater than splenic uptake (Fig. 5.8). The significance of suspicious focus of FDG uptake in the liver can be ascertained by checking whether the uptake is distinctly

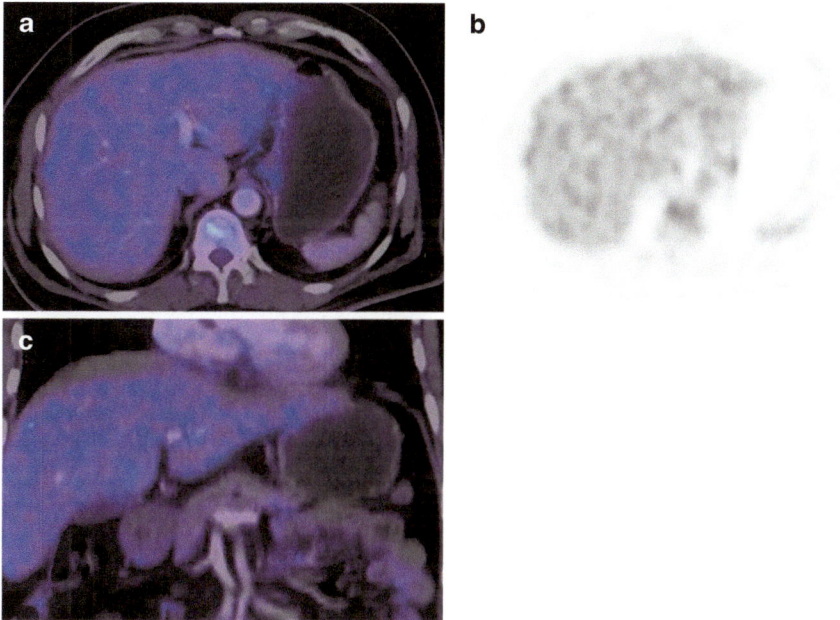

Fig. 5.8 Physiological FDG uptake in the liver (**a, c**). Fine mottled appearance of physiological FDG uptake in the liver made out in PET image

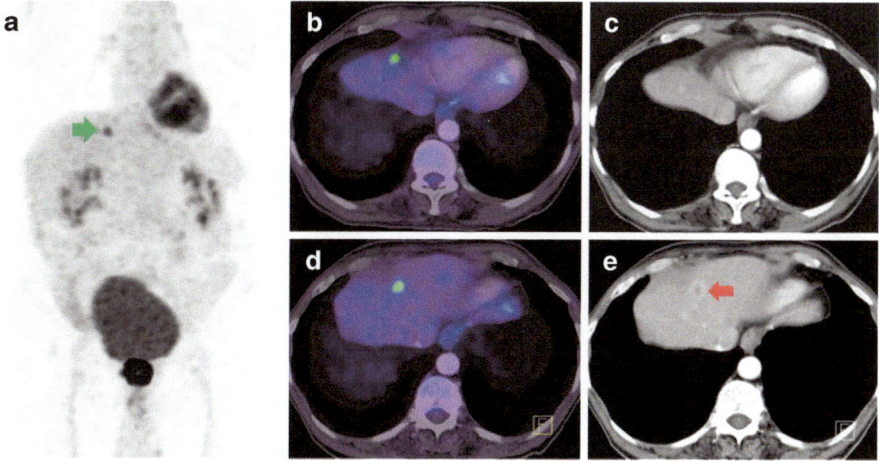

Fig. 5.9 Case of carcinoma of the rectum 18F-FDG PET/CT for initial staging reveals focal FDG uptake in the liver (**b**) with no corresponding lesion seen in CT part (**c**). Review of MIP shows the lesion to be significant (*green arrow*) (**a**). Movement misregistration is manually corrected, and corresponding CT image shows a peripherally contrast-enhancing lesion in segment VIII of the liver (*red arrow*) (**e**)

discernible in the maximum intensity projection image and whether there is a corresponding lesion in contrast-enhanced CT or MRI images (Fig. 5.9). False-positive and false-negative FDG uptake in the liver [11, 12] is described in Table 5.1.

Table 5.1 False-positive and false-negative FDG uptake in the liver with relevance to cases of colorectal malignancies

S. No.	False Negative	False positive
1	Lesions smaller than resolution of PET	Liver abscess
2	Necrotic and mucinous metastatic adenocarcinoma	Infarct
3	Post-chemotherapy	Granulomatous diseases
4	Coexistent hepatomas/infiltrative subtype of cholangiocarcinoma	Cholangitis (uptake along the biliary tree

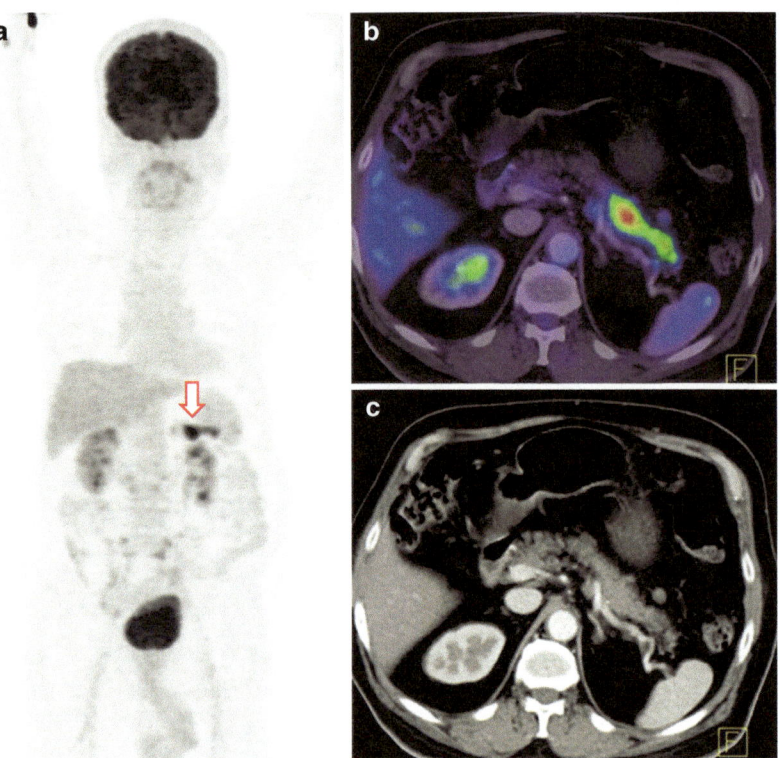

Fig. 5.10 A 73-year-old male patient who was a treated case of carcinoma of the rectum, on follow-up, mild rise in CEA levels was noted. 18F-FDG PET/CT (**a - MIP**) was done for suspected recurrence which showed abnormal intense FDG uptake on distal body and tail of pancreas (**b - axial fused PET/CT and c - axial contrast enhanced CT**) with no abnormal FDG avid lesions elsewhere in the body. CA19-9 levels were marked elevated. Distal pancreatectomy was done, and histopathology report revealed primary pancreatic adenocarcinoma

5.5.2 Spleen, Pancreas, and Adrenals

In general, splenic uptake greater than the liver is considered significant. Isolated focal increased FDG uptake in the pancreas in a case of colorectal malignancy is unlikely to be metastatic (Fig. 5.10). Increased FDG uptake (focal/diffusely increased) in the spleen [11], pancreas [13–14], and adrenals [15] is listed in Table 5.2.

Table 5.2 Causes of focal/diffusely increased FDG uptake in the spleen and pancreas

No.	Spleen	Pancreas	Adrenals
1.	Lymphoma	Primary pancreatic malignancy	Adenoma
2.	Myeloproliferative disorders	Pancreatitis	Hyperplasia
3.	Sarcoidosis	Post-radiation changes	Oncocytoma
4.	Infections—tuberculosis, kala-azar, malaria, infectious mononucleosis, etc.	Portal vein thrombus	Angiomyolipoma
5.	Chemotherapy	Haemorrhagic pseudocysts	Pheochromocytoma
6.	Exogenous marrow stimulation	Retroperitoneal fibrosis	Paraganglioma
7.	Metastasis	Metastasis	Metastasis

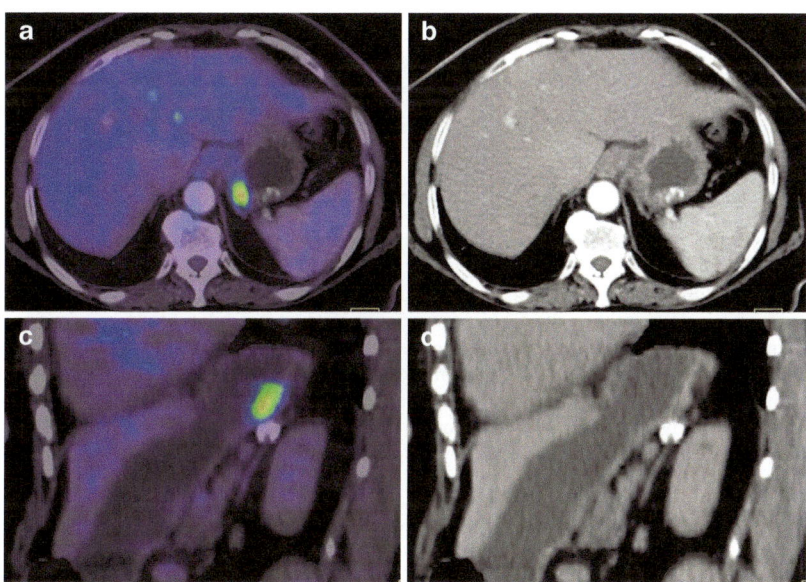

Fig. 5.11 IIncidentally detected FDG uptake in the posterior wall of cardia of the stomach (**a - axial fused PET/CT, b - axial contrast enhanced CT, c - coronal fused PET/CT and d - coronal contrast enhanced CT sections**). Upper GI endoscopy revealed a gastric ulcer, and biopsy was negative for malignancy

5.5.3   Stomach

Diffuse FDG uptake is often seen associated with gastritis. Focal FDG uptake in stomach if clinically significant can be further evaluated with endoscopy (Fig. 5.11).

5.5.4   Colon and Small Bowel

Oral contrast is particularly useful in characterising small bowel pathology and is routinely used in FDG PET/CT; however, rectal contrast is not routinely used.

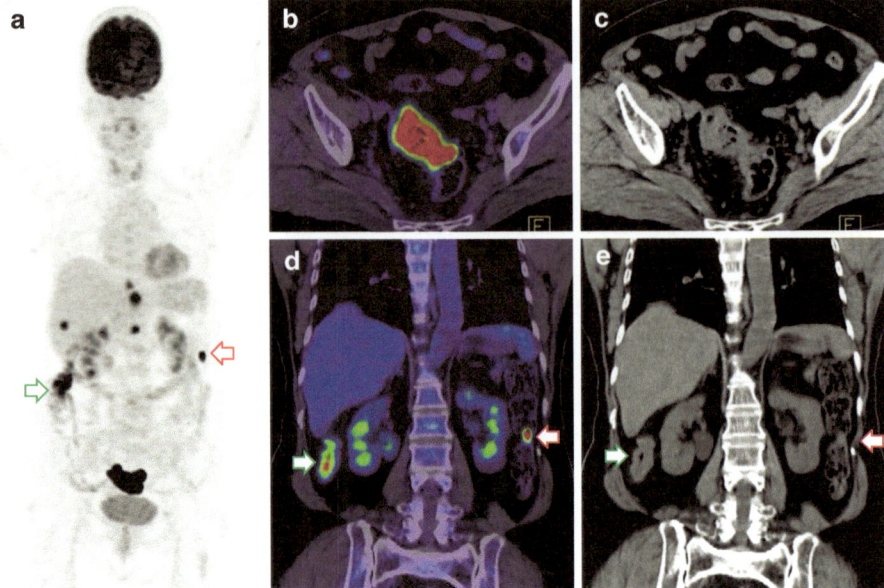

Fig. 5.12 A 71-year-old female with diagnosed carcinoma of the sigmoid colon, 18F-FDG PET/CT (**a - MIP**) for initial staging showed intense FDG uptake in the sigmoid colon (**b - fused PET/CT axial section, c - contrast enhanced CT axial section**). Focal abnormal intense FDG uptake (*red arrow*) was also noted in the middescending colon which turned out to be a neoplastic polyp (**d - coronal fused PET/CT, e - coronal contrast enhanced CT section**). A short segment of intense FDG uptake is noted in the ascending colon (*green arrow*) with apparent thickening in the unprepared bowel which did not correspond to any abnormality on colonoscopy. Significant FDG uptake in relatively long segments of the colon with no definite mural thickening on CT is often noted without any subsequent abnormality being identified

Careful correlation with adjunct CT findings is crucial in interpretation of FDG avidity in the colon (Fig. 5.12). Mostly characteristic CT findings help in identifying non-malignant causes of FDG uptake in the colon including appendicitis, diverticulitis, and focal abdominal or pelvic abscesses. Focal intense FDG activity in the colon (Fig. 5.13) may represent neoplastic lesion in up to 68% cases and hence warrants further evaluation with colonoscopy or CT colonography [16]. Intense large and small bowel uptake may be seen in diabetic patients on metformin (Fig. 5.14) [17].

5.5.5   Urinary Tract

Focal pooling of the tracer in the renal calyces or pelvis, dilated or redundant ureters, or bladder diverticula can mimic pelvic or retroperitoneal lymph node metastasis (Fig. 5.15). Careful review of the MIP image for the characteristic course of ureteric activity and search for coexistent anatomical lesion on CT part are helpful. The use of loop diuretics and delayed imaging helps to tackle the effects of radioactive urine in the urinary tract.

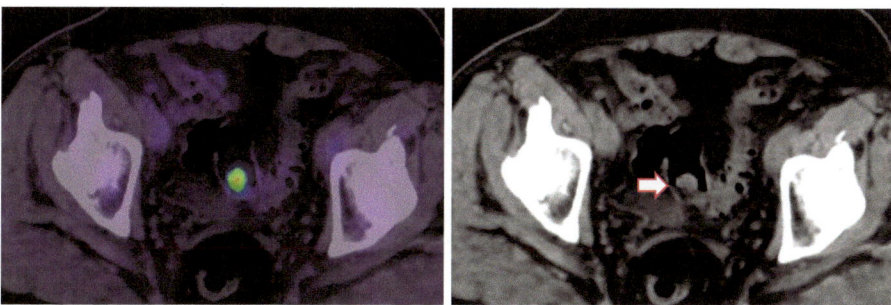

Fig. 5.13 Incidentally detected intense FDG uptake in a sigmoid polyp (*red arrow*), which on colonoscopy and biopsy was found to be malignant

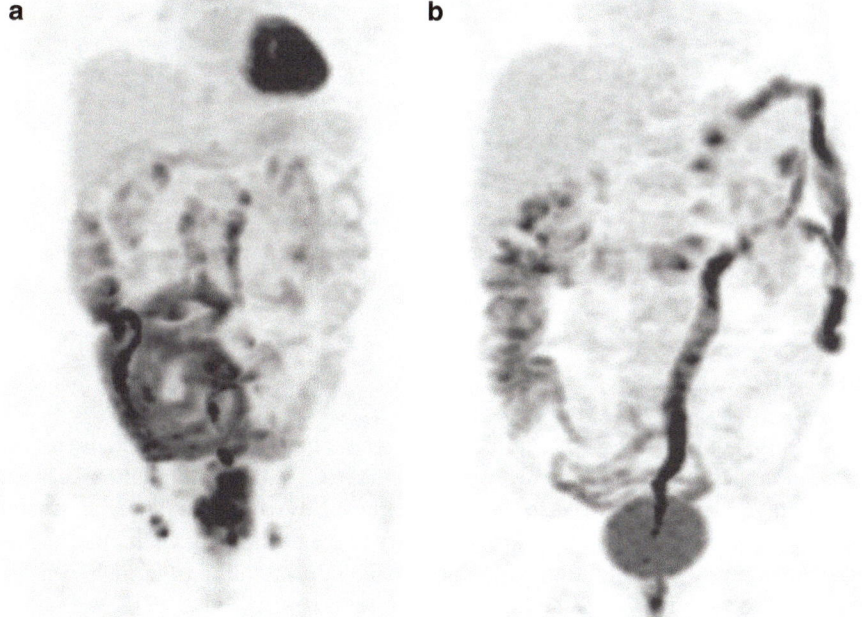

Fig. 5.14 High FDG uptake in bowel in patients on metformin

5.5.6   Reproductive System

In females, ovaries as well as uterus show variable physiological uptake depending on the phase of menstrual cycle. In males, prostate and testis may show variable physiological FDG uptake. Correlative anatomical imaging is helpful.

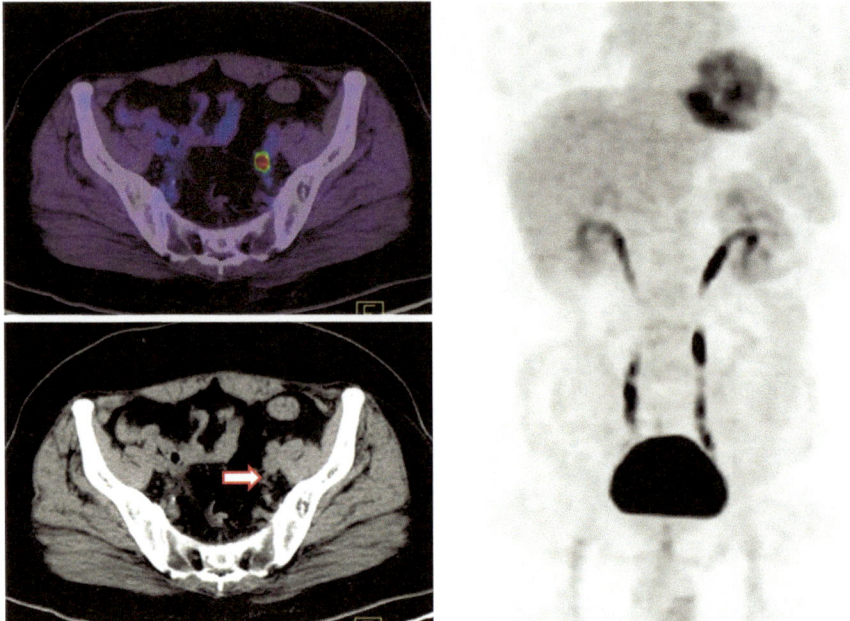

Fig. 5.15 Ureteric pooling of tracer mimicking FDG avid lymph node in fused PET/CT images. Review of CT images confirms the absence of lymph node (*red arrow*), and review of MIP images reveals the characteristic pattern of urinary activity in ureter on both sides

5.5.7 Bone

Bone lesions in the context of colorectal carcinoma have to be interpreted with caution. Sclerosis/lytic changes may not be obvious in CT; also benign mimickers with FDG uptake like Paget's disease (Fig. 5.16), fibrous dysplasia, and healing fracture exist. Diffuse increase in bone marrow activity is seen following chemotherapy and exogenous marrow stimulation which may make interpretation of bone lesions difficult. Diffuse marrow metastases, although rare, do exist (Fig. 5.17).

5.5.8 Muscle

Muscle metastases/deposits although rare have to be kept in mind (Fig. 5.18), and mimickers include abscess. Often tissue diagnosis is required in such cases especially in the context of cystic muscle metastases. Enthesitis can result in focal FDG uptake at the site of muscle insertion (Fig. 5.19).

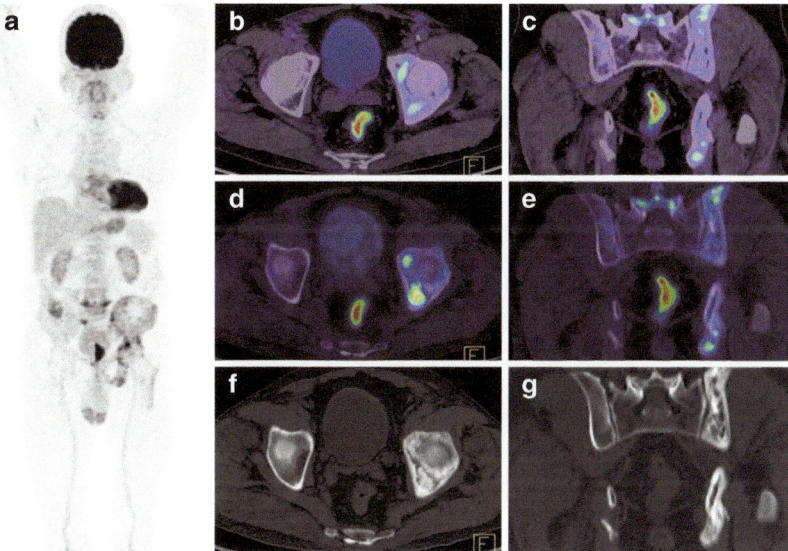

Fig. 5.16 A 68-year-old man with moderately differentiated adenocarcinoma of the rectum, 18FFDG PET/CT (**a - MIP**) for initial staging reveals intensely FDG-concentrating wall thickening in the rectum (**b, c**) with moderate patchy FDG uptake in diffuse sclerotic lesions (**d–g**) involving the left hemi pelvis and L5 vertebra. Biopsy from left iliac crest revealed it to be a Paget's disease

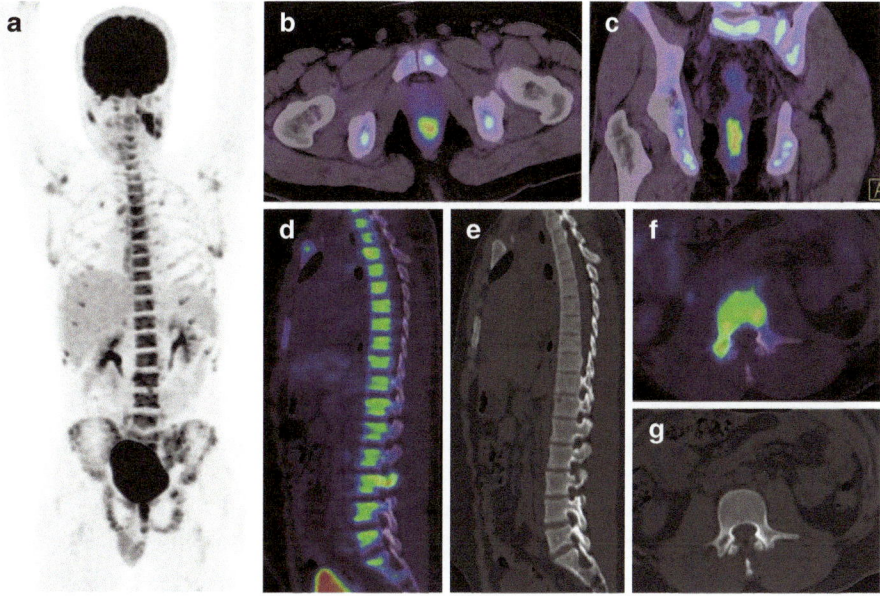

Fig. 5.17 A 28-year-old gentleman diagnosed with primary adenocarcinoma of the rectum, 18FFDG PET/CT (**a - MIP**) for initial staging showed intense FDG avid lesion in rectum (**b - axial fused PET/CT, c - coronal fused PET/CT**) with diffuse intense heterogeneous FDG uptake in the marrow (**d - sagittal fused PET/CT, e- sagittal CT section in bone window**). Heterogeneous FDG uptake in the marrow with involvement of the right pedicle of L3 vertebra (**f, g**), a bone marrow biopsy was done which confirmed marrow metastases from poorly differentiated adenocarcinoma

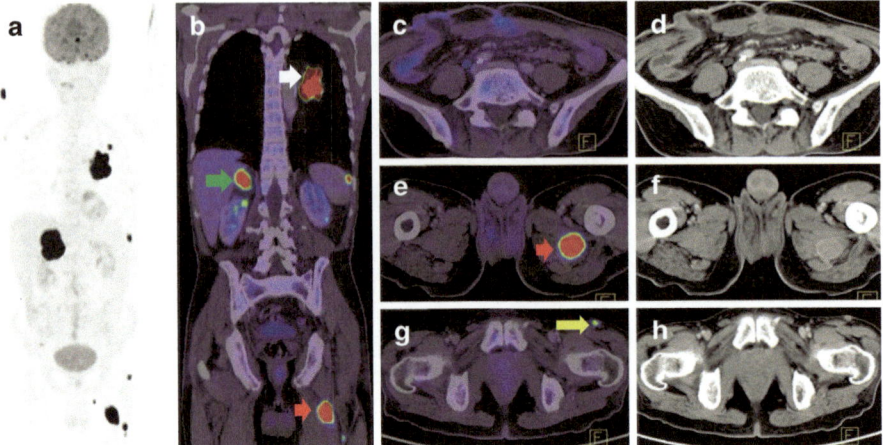

Fig. 5.18 A 64-year-old male patient diagnosed with adenocarcinoma of colon post-surgery and adjuvant chemotherapy, 18F-FDG PET/CT revealed no abnormal lesion in residual bowel (**c,d**); intensely FDG-concentrating mass lesion in the left hilar region (*white arrow*), right adrenal lesion (*green arrow*), skin nodule (*yellow arrow*), and muscle lesions (*red arrow*). Biopsy from the muscle lesion proved it to be metastatic adenocarcinoma, and second primary in the lung was later confirmed

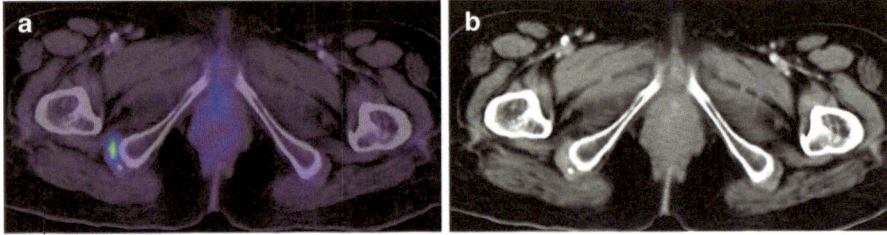

Fig. 5.19 Mild focal FDG uptake at the site of muscle attachment in the right ischium due to enthesitis

5.5.9 Lymph Nodes

An advantage of FDG PET is the ability to depict malignant neoplasms in lymph nodes when the nodes are not pathologically enlarged. False negatives include small-sized lymph nodes (smaller than the resolution of PET scanner), mucinous adenocarcinoma metastases, and post-chemotherapy. False positives include active granulomatous disease such as tuberculosis and sarcoidosis and infection or recent instrumentation resulting in high FDG uptake in involved nodes (Fig. 5.20) [11]. In cases of colorectal malignancies, isolated mediastinal/cervical lymph nodal FDG uptake in the absence of abdominal and pelvic disease should be considered as unrelated to colorectal malignancy unless otherwise proved (Fig. 5.21).

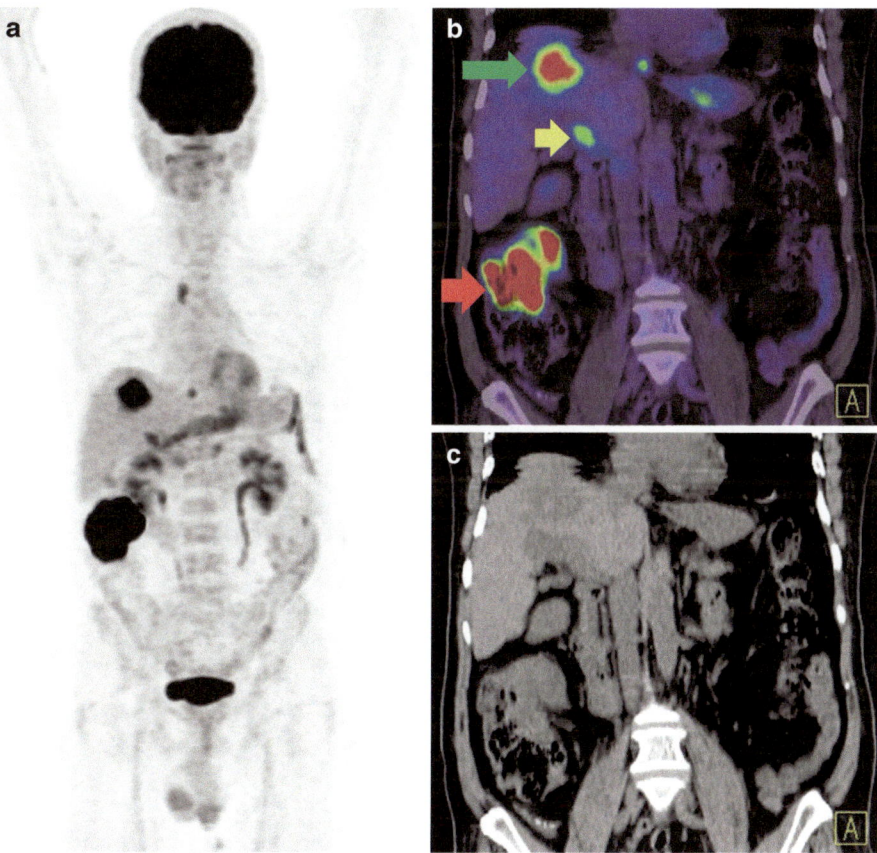

Fig. 5.20 A 75-year-old man with carcinoma in the ascending colon and suspected liver metastasis in segment VIII on contrast-enhanced CT abdomen underwent 18F-FDG PET/CT which showed intensely FDG-concentrating primary lesion in the ascending colon (*red arrow*), intensely FDG-concentrating lesion in segment VIII (*green arrow*), and moderately FDG-concentrating lesion in periportal lymph node (*yellow arrow*). Right hemicolectomy with metastasectomy of liver lesion and lymph nodal dissection was done, with final histopathology confirming adenocarcinoma of the ascending colon and with liver abscess and reactive periportal lymph node

5.5.10 Peritoneum

Increased FDG uptake is frequently seen in peritoneal metastases which appear either nodular or diffuse (Fig. 5.22). The peritoneal disease may not be associated with any abnormal FDG uptake in small-volume disease. False-positive FDG uptake may also be seen in the peritoneum postoperatively due to inflammation. Malignant ascites does not take up FDG.

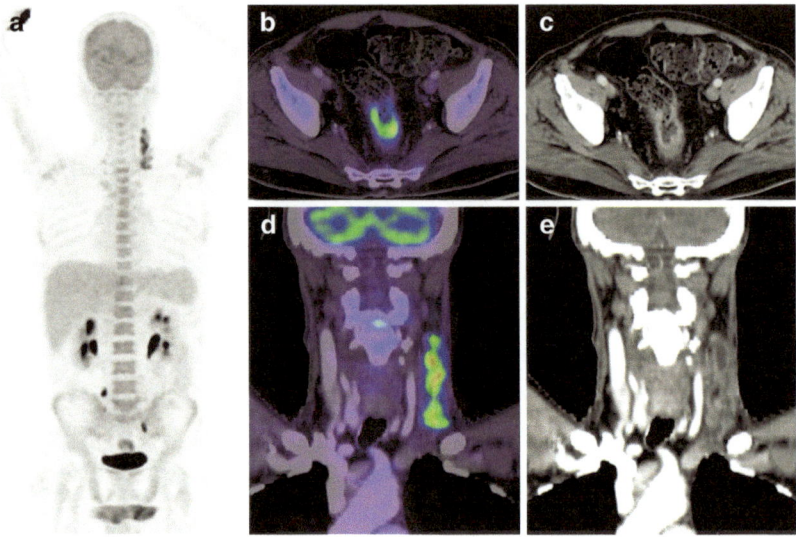

Fig. 5.21 A 53-year-old man diagnosed with carcinoma of the rectum, 18F-FDG PET/CT (**a - MIP**) for initial staging revealed intense FDG uptake in the primary lesion in rectum (**b, c**). There was no evidence of any pelvic or abdominal lymphadenopathy. Intensely FDG-concentrating necrotic left cervical lymph nodes were noted (**d, e**). Biopsy of the cervical lymph nodes confirmed it to be due to tuberculous lymphadenopathy

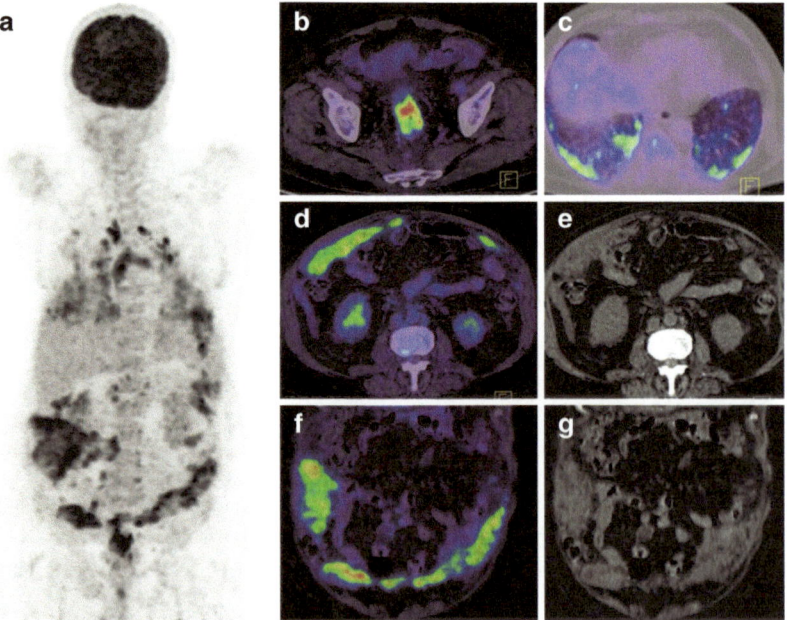

Fig. 5.22 A 66-year-old man with carcinoma of the rectosigmoid, 18F FDG PET/CT shows intense FDG avid primary site (**b**), extensive intensely FDG-avid omental nodules and omental thickening (**d–f**) with FDG avid lung lesions (**c**) and mediastinal lymph nodes

5.6   Treatment-Related Pitfalls

Surgery, radiation therapy, and chemotherapy forms an integral part of the treatment plan of colorectal malignancies. False-positive FDG uptake following surgery and radiation therapy can occur unless adequate time gap is given with the PET/CT. False negative (no uptake in scan with disease on histopathology) can be seen at primary site, lymph nodes, and liver lesions following chemotherapy. Postsurgical complications like haematoma and surgical abscesses can result in false-positive FDG uptake. Stoma/anastomotic sites can show diffuse or focal FDG uptake, and careful review of CT images for any abnormal thickening or mass lesions is required to clarify possibility of disease involvement (Fig. 5.23). Exogenous marrow stimulation or chemotherapy can result in increased FDG uptake in bone marrow which may make identification of skeletal lesions difficult (Fig. 5.24). Treatment for coexistent disease can also complicate interpretation of FDG avid lesions and requires judicial clinical judgement (Fig. 5.25).

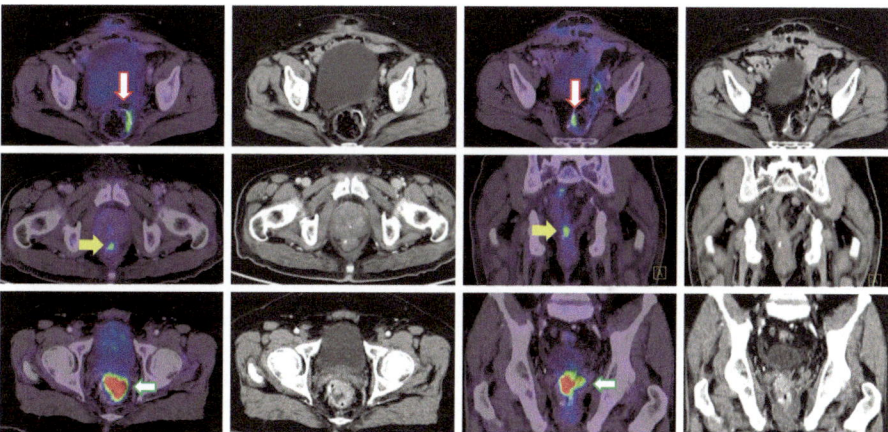

Fig. 5.23 Anastomotic site FDG uptake interpretation: Upper row images—FDG PET/CT scan done 4 weeks after surgery for restaging shows post-surgical inflammation (*red arrow*) with no abnormal wall thickening at the anastomotic site. Middle row images—FDG PET/CT scan done 2 years after surgery in a patient with rising CEA levels. Mild FDG uptake is noted at the anastomotic site with doubtful thickening (*yellow arrow*). Colonoscopy is suggested for further evaluation of the anastomotic site. Lower row images: FDG PET/CT scan done 1.5 years after surgery showing intensely FDG-concentrating definitive lesion at the anastomotic site (*green arrow*)

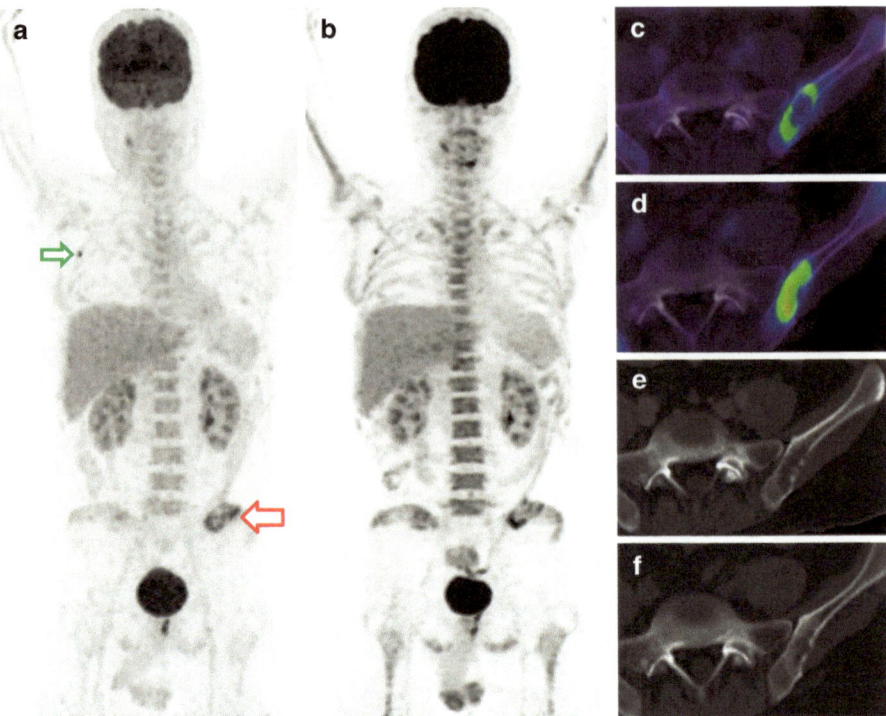

Fig. 5.24 A 56-year-old man who is a treated case of carcinoma of the rectum (surgery and adjuvant chemoradiation) on follow-up had rising CEA levels. 18F FDG PET/CT (**a - MIP**) for suspected recurrence evaluation revealed increased FDG uptake in the left iliac bone (*red arrow*) and right third rib (*green arrow*). Biopsy from left iliac bone confirmed the metastasis, and he underwent three cycles of chemotherapy. 18F-FDG PET/CT for response evaluation (**b**) shows diffuse FDG uptake in marrow due to reactive changes sparing the RT field in pelvis. Pretreatment FDG uptake in the left iliac bone (**c**), and corresponding lytic lesion (**e**) is noted. Careful observation and interpretation of findings are required as posttreatment FDG uptake is increased (**d**) with development of mild sclerotic changes in the left iliac bone lesion (**f**) and no new lesions are noted

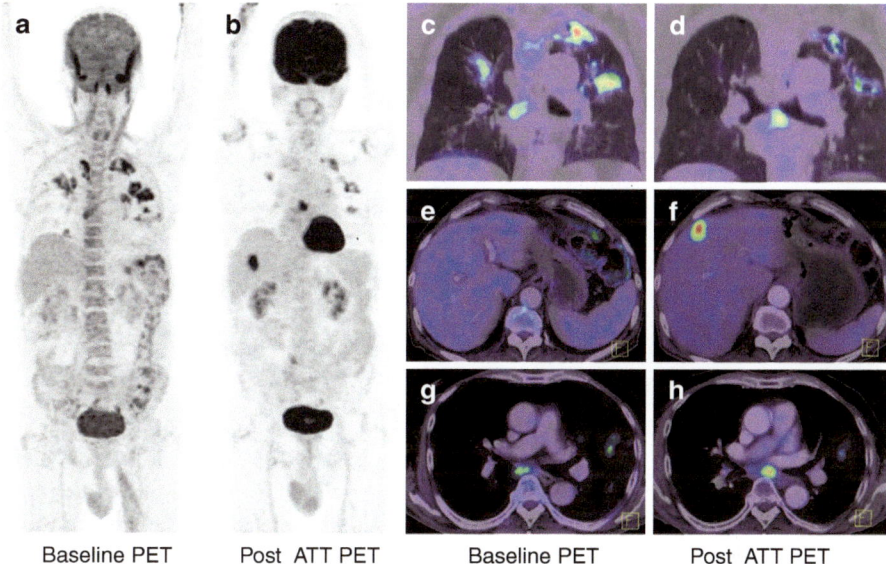

Baseline PET   Post ATT PET   Baseline PET   Post ATT PET

Fig. 5.25 A 66-year-old treated case of carcinoma of the rectum posttreatment on follow-up developed unexplained loss of weight and appetite with mild elevation of CEA levels. 18F-FDG PET/CT for suspected recurrence (**a - MIP**) revealed intensely FDG avid cavitary lesions in the upper lobe of both the lung fields (**c**) with FDG avid mediastinal lymph nodes (**g**). The presence of acid-fast bacilli was confirmed in bronchoalveolar lavage, and the patient was started on ATT. After completing 6 months of antitubercular treatment (ATT), 18F-FDG PET/CT (**b - MIP**) was repeated as the CEA levels rose significantly. Post-ATT PET showed reduction in FDG avidity in the lung lesions (**d**) and mediastinal lymph nodes except subcarinal lymph node which showed increase in FDG avidity (**h**). Intensely FDG-concentrating new lesion was noted in the liver (**e - baseline PET axial section with no liver lesion and f - corresponding section in follow up PET with liver lesion**) which was suspicious for liver metastasis and later on confirmed on biopsy and histopathology as metastasis

Conclusion

FDG PET/CT is a very useful tool in the management of colorectal malignancies. Careful elucidation of clinical history, minimising technical artefacts, and an adequate understanding of the physiological variants and imaging pitfalls of FDG PET/CT help in accurate reporting of FDG PET/CT in colorectal malignancies.

Key Points

- A thorough understanding of sites of physiological uptake in the abdomen and pelvis is an essential prerequisite to interpret FDG PET/CT scans in colorectal carcinoma.

- Respiratory motion artefacts predominantly affect structures close to the diaphragm especially liver lesions and basal lung lesions. Review of PET alone images and identification of any associated CT abnormalities would be helpful.

- Bowel peristalsis and positional changes also result in misregistration, particularly in the small bowel.

- Physiological FDG uptake in the liver is homogeneous/uniformly mottled and slightly greater than splenic uptake. The significance of suspicious focus of FDG uptake in the liver can be ascertained by checking whether the uptake is distinctly discernible in the maximum intensity projection image and whether there is a corresponding lesion in contrast-enhanced CT or MRI images.

- Diffuse FDG uptake is often seen associated with gastritis. Focal FDG uptake in the stomach if clinically significant can be further evaluated with endoscopy.

- Oral contrast is particularly useful in characterising small bowel pathology and is routinely used in FDG PET/CT; however, rectal contrast is not routinely used.

- Careful correlation with adjunct CT findings is crucial in interpretation of FDG avidity in the colon.

- Focal intense FDG activity in the colon may represent neoplastic lesion in up to 68% cases and hence warrants further evaluation with colonoscopy or CT colonography.

- Intense large and small bowel uptake may be seen in diabetic patients on metformin.

- Focal pooling of the tracer in the renal calyces or pelvis, dilated or redundant ureters, or bladder diverticula can mimic pelvic or retroperitoneal lymph node metastasis.

- Ovaries as well as uterus shows variable physiological uptake depending on the phase of menstrual cycle.

- False-positive FDG uptake following surgery and radiation therapy can occur unless adequate time gap is given with the PET/CT.

- False negative (no uptake in scan with disease on histopathology) can be seen at primary site, lymph nodes, and liver lesions following chemotherapy.

- Postsurgical complications like haematoma and surgical abscesses can result in false-positive FDG uptake.

- Stoma/anastomotic sites can show diffuse or focal FDG uptake, and careful review of CT images for any abnormal thickening or mass lesions is required to clarify possibility of disease involvement.

References

1. Laurens ST, Oyen WJ. Impact of fluorodeoxyglucose PET/computed tomography on the management of patients with colorectal cancer. PET Clin. 2015;10(3):345–60.
2. Petersen RK, Hess S, Alavi A, et al. Clinical impact of FDG-PET/CT on colorectal cancer staging and treatment strategy. Am J Nucl Med Mol Imaging. 2014;4(5):471–82.
3. Kostakoglu L, Hardoff R, Mirtcheva R, Goldsmith SJ. PET—CT fusion imaging in differentiating physiologic from pathologic FDG uptake. Radiographics. 2004;24(5):1411–31.
4. Kostakoglu L, Agress H, Goldsmith SJ. Clinical role of FDG PET in evaluation of cancer patients. Radiographics. 2003;23:315–39.
5. Blake MA, Singh A, Setty BN, et al. Pearls and pitfalls in interpretation of abdominal and pelvic PETCT. Radiographics. 2006;26(5):1335–53.
6. Emmott J, Sanghera B, Chambers J, Wong WL. The effects of Nbutylscopolamine on bowel uptake: an 18FFDG PET study. Nucl Med Commun. 2008;29(1):11–6.
7. Corrigan AJ, Schleyer PJ, Cook GJ. Pitfalls and artifacts in the use of PET/CT in oncology imaging. Semin Nucl Med. 2015;45(6):481–99.
8. Kapoor V, McCook BM, Torok FS. An introduction to PET CT imaging. Radiographics. 2004;24(2):523–43.
9. Sureshbabu W, Mawlawi O. PET/CT imaging artifacts. J Nucl Med Technol. 2005;33(3):156–61. quiz 63–64
10. Mawlawi O, Erasmus JJ, Pan T, et al. Truncation artifact on PET/CT: impact on measurements of activity concentration and assessment of a correction algorithm. AJR Am J Roentgenol. 2006;186(5):1458–67.
11. McDermott S, Skehan SJ. Whole body imaging in the abdominal cancer patient: pitfalls of PET-CT. Abdom Imaging. 2010;35(1):55–69.
12. Donadon M, Bona S, Montorsi M, et al. FDG-PET positive granuloma of the liver mimicking local recurrence after hepatic resection of colorectal liver metastasis. Hepato-Gastroenterology. 2010;57:138–9.
13. Bares R, Klever P, Hauptmann S, et al. F18 fluorodeoxyglucose PET in vivo evaluation of pancreatic glucose metabolism for detection of pancreatic cancer. Radiology. 1994;192(1):79–86.
14. Friess H, Langhans J, Ebert M, et al. Diagnosis of pancreatic cancer by [18F] fluoro-2-deoxy-d-glucose positron emission tomography. Gut. 1995;36(5):771–7.
15. Culverwell AD, Scarsbrook AF, Chowdhury FU. False-positive uptake on 2-[18F]-fluoro-2-deoxy-D-glucose(FDG)positron-emission tomog- raphy/computed tomography(PET/CT) in oncological imaging. Clin Radiol. 2011;66:366–82.

16. Treglia G, Taralli S, Salsano M, et al. Prevalence and malignancy risk of focal colorectal inci-
    dental uptake detected by 18F-FDG-PETorPET/CT: a meta-analysis. Radiol Oncol.
    2014;48(2):99–104.
17. Gontier E, Fourme E, Wartski M, et al. High and typical 18F-FDG bowel uptake in patients
    treated with metformin. Eur J Nucl Med Mol Imaging. 2008;35:95–9.

PET/CT in Colorectal Cancer

6

Yong Du

Contents

6.1   Introduction

Colorectal cancer, also called bowel cancer, is the third most common cancer in both males (14% of the male total) and females (11%) in the UK. In 2011, there were 41,581 new cases of bowel cancer in the UK. It is the second most common cause of cancer death in the UK, accounting for 10% of all deaths from cancer. The overall predicted 5-year survival rate is 59% for patients diagnosed with bowel cancer during 2010–2011 in England and Wales. Worldwide, it is also the third most common cancer, with more than 1,360,000 new cases diagnosed in 2012 (10% of the total).

Bowel cancer mortality rates have decreased overall in the UK and Europe since the 1970s, likely owing to the earlier detection and improved treatment. Over the last decade, European age-standardised mortality rates have decreased by 15% in males and 12% in females with colorectal cancer. Nonetheless, the burden of the

Y. Du, M.B.B.S., M.Sc., Ph.D., F.R.C.P.
Department of Nuclear Medicine and PET/CT, Royal Marsden NHS
Foundation Trust, London, UK
e-mail: yong.du@rmh.nhs.uk

© Springer International Publishing Switzerland 2017   49
Y. Du (ed.), *PET/CT in Colorectal Cancer*, Clinicians' Guides to Radionuclide
Hybrid Imaging - PET/CT, DOI 10.1007/978-3-319-54837-1_6

Table 6.1 Clinical indications for [18]FDG-PET/CT in colorectal cancer

	[18]FDG-PET/CT indications	Interpretation
Staging/diagnosis	Not routinely required Should be performed if CT detected synchronous liver metastases and patient is considered for radical treatment Should be performed if CT or MRI detected common iliac nodal metastases Should be considered if CT detected equivocal metastatic lesions	Lesions demonstrate increased metabolic activity
Restaging/response assessment	Not routinely required Should be considered if avoidance of surgery is considered or indeterminate on conventional imaging such as CT or MRI	Reassessment [18]FDG-PET/CT should be interpreted with consideration of patients' clinical history including prior chemoradiation, local targeted therapy such as RFA or surgical history
Detection of recurrence	Should be performed in patients with recurrent disease being considered for radical treatment Should be performed in patients with rising tumour markers and/or being clinically suspicious of recurrence but with negative or equivocal findings on other imaging Assessment of indeterminate presacral mass	[18]FDG-PET/CT study should be interpreted with consideration of patients' clinical history including chemoradiation, local targeted therapy such as RFA or surgical history

disease and mortality is still high, and further improvement in diagnostic accuracy including tumour-node-metastasis (TNM) staging and tumour biology characterisation remains essential for a better selection of treatment approaches by an experienced multidisciplinary expert team [1–3]. In addition to conventional morphological imaging modalities such as CT, ultrasound and MRI, [18]FDG-PET/CT plays instrumental roles in several areas critical for the optimal management of colorectal cancer, as summarised in Table 6.1 and discussed in detail below.

6.2   Primary Diagnosis/Staging

For routine staging of colon or rectal cancer, complete colonoscopy and CT of the chest and abdomen are required. In addition, pelvic MRI should be performed for all rectal cancer patients for better local disease delineation [2].

[18]FDG-PET/CT is not required unless CT detects synchronous liver metastases, and the patient could be considered for curative liver surgery as [18]FDG-PET/CT is more sensitive than CT to rule out extrahepatic metastases. [18]FDG-PET/CT should

also be performed if staging CT or MRI scan detects nodal metastases in the common iliac region or equivocal findings such as indeterminate pulmonary, liver or bony lesions.

[18]FDG-PET/CT is not required if other imaging modality, for example, CT, has already demonstrated widespread metastatic disease and the patient would not be eligible for radical treatment [2].

6.3 Response Assessment

As discussed in the previous chapter, Management of Colorectal Cancer, surgery is the mainstay of treatment of localised colorectal cancer. However, the treatment of low and mid rectal cancer (up to 10 cm distance of the anal verge) differs greatly from that of colon or sigmoid cancers. Whilst surgery for local control of disease in colonic cancer is more feasible, resection of mid and low rectal cancer is much more challenging as the surgery would be restricted by several factors due to the anatomical location of the rectum. In particular, from a surgical as well as post-surgery quality of life point of view, it is always of importance to preserve the sphincter function, if possible, and to maintain the genitourinary function. As a result, for colonic cancer, adjuvant chemotherapy is usually recommended only for locally advanced colon cancer patients after surgery, but neoadjuvant chemo-radiation would be given to all patients with mid- or low rectal cancer to downstage the tumour so as to reduce the risk of local relapse, improve the chance of R0 resection, preserve sphincter function, avoid stoma or even avoid surgery in selected patients especially if a pathological complete response could be confirmed.

To assess response to treatment, currently, none of the imaging modalities (ERUS, MRI, CT) can reliably predict a complete remission. Although downsizing can be assessed with those imaging technologies, accuracy for pathological T staging and regression rate/histopathological response is low owing to multiple factors, fundamentally due to the inability of any of these imaging techniques to detect microscopic disease [2].

Recent studies suggested diffusion-weighted MRI might be more sensitive than MRI only in predicting a pathological complete response but still with limited accuracy. Similarly, the role of [18]FDG-PET/CT in this setting is also under investigation. Several ongoing studies are testing if [18]FDG-PET/CT is any better than MRI and/or if the combination of [18]FDG-PET/CT and MRI could be more reliable than each modality alone (Fig. 6.1) [4–11].

In line with the advancement of radiotherapy techniques, another area of clinical interest is if advanced imaging technologies such as functional MRI or PET/CT with either [18]FDG or other tracers such as [18]FLT or [18]FMISO could help identify relatively radioresistant tumour components so as to local intensification of radiotherapy could be deployed to achieve higher rates of disease control without unacceptable toxicity.

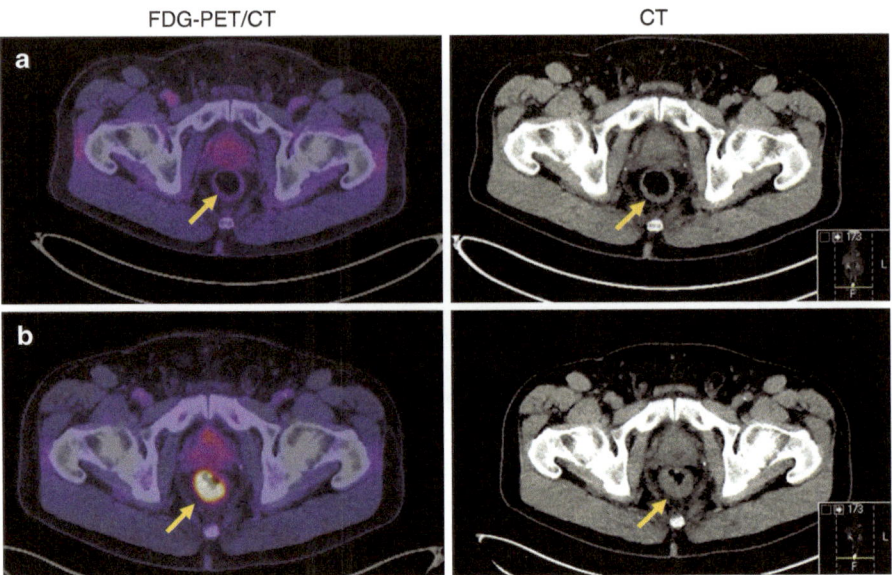

Fig. 6.1 [18]FDG-PET/CT performed 4 weeks after neoadjuvant chemoradiation demonstrates a true complete pathological response in a low rectal cancer patient

6.4   Detection of Recurrent Disease

[18]FDG-PET/CT has demonstrated higher sensitivity than conventional imaging (CT or MRI) in detecting systemic metastatic disease. It therefore should be performed in patients with recurrent disease being considered for radical treatment and/or metastasectomy to avoid futile invasive interventions.

Likewise, [18]FDG-PET/CT should also be performed in patients with rising tumour markers (e.g. CEA) and/or being clinically suspicious of recurrence but with negative or equivocal findings on other imaging.

Another indication for [18]FDG-PET/CT is to evaluate the nature of post-surgery presacral masses. It is a common feature for patients to present with persistent presacral soft tissue mass after radical resection of rectal cancer. On conventional morphological imaging, such masses could be variable in size and morphological appearances and therefore difficult to tell on CT if active tumour grows within the mass until it has grown significantly.

6.5   Normal Variants and Artefacts

Compared to the old days when [18]FDG-PET studies were performed on stand-alone PET scanners, the advent of modern hybrid PET/CT technology at the beginning of the twenty-first century has made the recognition of non-cancerous variants much easier. However, several usual artefacts as summarised in Table 6.2 should always be born in mind when interpreting a routine [18]FDG-PET/CT study.

Table 6.2 Normal variants and artefacts on [18]FDG-PET/CT in colorectal cancer

Normal variants and artefacts	[18]FDG-PET/CT imaging features
Non-specific bowel uptake	Variable, usually low-grade, diffuse uptake along the large bowel; can be high-grade uptake on metformin in diabetic patients but with no corresponding mural thickening on CT images of the PET/CT study
Diverticulitis	Variable but always associated with diverticular disease on CT images of the PET/CT study
Mucinous cancer	[18]FDG uptake could be variable but usually relatively low grade in mucinous cancer and therefore low sensitivity in detecting such cancers
Urinary activity	Usually can be readily recognised with the aid of corresponding CT images of the modern PET/CT study but can be difficult in lean patients or in post-surgery patients due to the disturbed anatomy
Presacral mass	Non-cancerous presacral mass usually has very low-grade [18]FDG avidity, but if it contains active inflammatory component which are usually very [18]FDG avid, it could be very difficult to differentiate inflammation from tumour involvement. Interval re-scan or biopsy could be required

Non-specific Bowel Uptake: Another physiological variant is non-specific smooth muscle uptake of [18]FDG by the bowel wall. Although the appearances of such non-specific uptake could be highly variable but differing from bowel cancer, they are usually diffuse, and the uptake is usually relatively low grade. With the aid of the CT component of the modern hybrid [18]FDG-PET/CT, it is usually not difficult to recognise such physiological uptake as it would present with no corresponding bowel wall mural thickening, a typical feature for a bowel cancer.

Diabetic Patients: Particular attention should be made to diabetic patients as antidiabetic medication such as metformin usually leads to significantly increased [18]FDG uptake by the large bowel. This variant can be readily recognised in correlation with patients' medication history, and in addition, such uptake is usually also diffuse, along much of the large bowel, with no mural thickening.

Diverticulitis: Sometimes, active large bowel diverticulitis also leads to focal or diffuse increased [18]FDG uptake. This variant can be better identified with the aid of the CT component of the PET/CT study.

Mucinous Cancer: [18]FDG is known to have low avidity in mucinous or signet ring cancers which consist of approximately 10–15% of colorectal cancers, largely due to the low tumour cellularity and abundant mucin within such tumours. In a retrospective observation reported by Berger et al., [18]FDG-PET detected only 59% (13 out of 22) mucinous cancer.

Urinary Activity: [18]FDG is physiologically excreted by the urinary system. Aided by the corresponding CT images of the modern PET/CT study, it is usually not difficult to identify the urinary tract, but sometimes, it can be difficult to differentiate small-volume retroperitoneal nodal uptake from nearby ureteric activity; sometimes, it could also be difficult to identify the boundary of the rectal primary from the adjacent bladder especially when there is locally advanced rectal primary invading into adjacent structures. In such cases, corresponding with contrast-enhanced CT or pelvic MRI scans might be beneficial.

Presacral Mass: As discussed above, in rectal cancer patients, it is a usual feature to develop non-specific post-surgical presacral soft tissue masses. In most cases, the mass is consisted of fibrotic tissue secondary to post-surgical inflammatory process. Such soft tissue is usually ill-defined and fairly small volume and could gradually reduce in size with time. However, local recurrence is unfortunately a common problem in rectal cancer usually involving the presacral region. [18]FDG-PET/CT has distinctive advantage in the early differentiation of active tumour from a chronic fibrotic process as the later would be either [18]FDG negative or showing very low-grade diffuse uptake, whilst the former usually demonstrates focal or irregular high-grade [18]FDG uptake. The only pitfall is, however, when the presacral mass contains active inflammatory elements, sometimes but not always, associated with fistulation.

Timing of 18FDG-PET/CT Scanning: [18]FDG-PET/CT should be performed routinely at least 4 weeks after surgery or completion of chemoradiation to avoid the contamination from active post-surgical inflammatory changes as well as local inflammation following radiotherapy which could mimic active residual disease. On the same note, even if the scan was performed long after surgical or other therapeutic intervention, there is always low-grade non-specific physiological [18]FDG uptake along the bowel wall. This would inevitably render it extremely difficult to rule out any small-volume residual disease on a [18]FDG-PET/CT study. Although in experienced eyes, non-specific low-grade uptake can be readily recognised, it is currently the limitations of any clinical imaging technology, including [18]FDG-PET/CT, to detect or rule out microscopic disease.

Key Points

- In addition to conventional morphological imaging modalities such as CT, ultrasound and MRI, [18]FDG-PET/CT plays instrumental roles in several areas critical for the optimal management of colorectal cancer.

Primary Diagnosis/Staging

- [18]FDG-PET/CT is not required unless CT detects synchronous liver metastases and the patient could be considered for curative liver surgery.

- [18]FDG-PET/CT should also be performed if staging CT or MRI scan detects nodal metastases or equivocal findings such as indeterminate pulmonary, liver or bony lesions.

Response Assessment

- Recent studies suggested diffusion-weighted MRI might be more sensitive than MRI only in predicting a pathological complete response but still with limited accuracy. Similarly, the role of [18]FDG-PET/CT in this setting is also under investigation.

Detection of Recurrent Disease

- ^{18}FDG-PET/CT has demonstrated higher sensitivity than conventional imaging (CT or MRI) in detecting systemic metastatic disease.

- ^{18}FDG-PET/CT should also be performed in patients with rising tumour markers and/or being clinically suspicious of recurrence but with negative or equivocal findings on other imaging.

- ^{18}FDG-PET/CT is used to evaluate the nature of post-surgery presacral masses.

References

1. DeSantis CE, Lin CC, Mariotto AB, et al. Cancer treatment and survivorship statistics, 2014. CA Cancer J Clin. 2014;64:252–71.
2. Schmoll HJ, Van CE, Stein A, et al. ESMO consensus guidelines for management of patients with colon and rectal cancer. A personalized approach to clinical decision making. Ann Oncol. 2012;23:2479–516.
3. Siegel R, DeSantis C, Jemal A. Colorectal cancer statistics, 2014. CA Cancer J Clin. 2014;64:104–17.
4. Berger KL, Nicholson SA, Dehdashti F, et al. FDG PET evaluation of mucinous neoplasms: correlation of FDG uptake with histopathologic features. AJR Am J Roentgenol. 2000;174:1005–8.
5. Brush J, Boyd K, Chappell F, et al. The value of FDG positron emission tomography/computerised tomography (PET/CT) in pre-operative staging of colorectal cancer: a systematic review and economic evaluation. Health Technol Assess. 2011;15:1–192.
6. Lastoria S, Piccirillo MC, Caraco C, et al. Early PET/CT scan is more effective than RECIST in predicting outcome of patients with liver metastases from colorectal cancer treated with preoperative chemotherapy plus bevacizumab. J Nucl Med. 2013;54:2062–9.
7. Maizlin ZV, Brown JA, So G, et al. Can CT replace MRI in preoperative assessment of the circumferential resection margin in rectal cancer? Dis Colon rectum. 2010;53:308–14.
8. Perez RO, Habr-Gama A, Gama-Rodrigues J, et al. Accuracy of positron emission tomography/computed tomography and clinical assessment in the detection of complete rectal tumor regression after neoadjuvant chemoradiation: long-term results of a prospective trial (National Clinical Trial 00254683). Cancer. 2012;118:3501–11.
9. Siriwardena AK, Mason JM, Mullamitha S, et al. Management of colorectal cancer presenting with synchronous liver metastases. Nat Rev Clin Oncol. 2014;11:446–59.
10. Stein A, Hiemer S, Schmoll HJ. Adjuvant therapy for early colon cancer: current status. Drugs. 2011;71:2257–75.
11. Tagliabue L. The emerging role of FDG PET/CT in rectal cancer management: is it time to use the technique for early prognostication? Eur J Nucl Med Mol Imaging. 2013;40:652–6.

PET/CT in Colorectal Cancer-Pictorial Atlas

7

Yong Du

Contents

Y. Du, M.B.B.S., M.Sc., Ph.D., F.R.C.P.
Department of Nuclear Medicine and PET/CT, Royal Marsden NHS Foundation Trust,
London, UK
e-mail: yong.du@rmh.nhs.uk

© Springer International Publishing Switzerland 2017   57
Y. Du (ed.), *PET/CT in Colorectal Cancer*, Clinicians' Guides to Radionuclide
Hybrid Imaging - PET/CT, DOI 10.1007/978-3-319-54837-1_7

7.1   Case 1: Typical "Apple-Core" Appearance on CT of a Transverse Colon Primary. CT Staging: T3N2M0

Clinical details: A 9-year-old female presented with positive FOB; colonoscopy found impassable stricture at the transverse colon. CT scan demonstrates an approximately 3.5 cm annular lesions within the transverse colon as illustrated below.

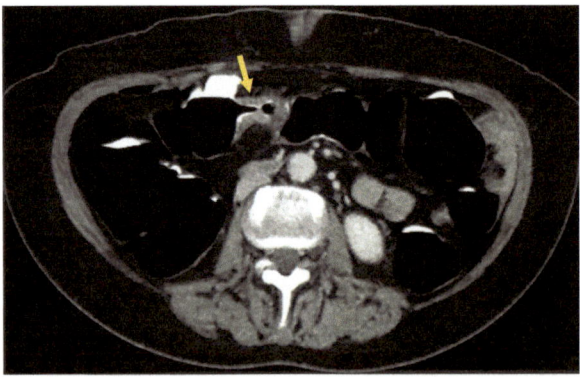

Teaching points: CT scan is the primary imaging modality for staging colon cancer, alongside colonoscopy. The typical appearance of a colon cancer is usually described as an "apple core" due to the tumour-associated bowel wall thickening/ stricture as illustrated in this case.

7.2   Case 2: Sigmoid Colon Primary. CT Staging: T3N2M0

Clinical details: A 74-year-old male presented with positive FOB; colonoscopy found mass lesion in the sigmoid colon, and biopsy confirmed moderately differentiated adenocarcinoma. CT scan demonstrates an approximately 5 cm annular lesions within the sigmoid colon as illustrated below.

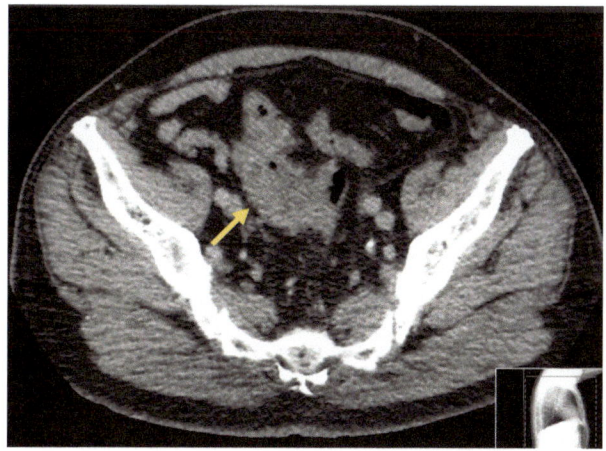

   Teaching points: CT scan is the primary imaging modality for staging colon cancer, alongside colonoscopy. The typical appearance of a colon cancer is demonstrated here with circumferential mural thickening of the affected segment of the bowel loop.

7.3   Case 3: Adenocarcinoma Within the Splenic Flexure of the Colon. On CT, the Approximately 5 cm Annular Lesion Is in Close Contact with the Anterior Surface and the Upper Pole of the Left Kidney as Illustrated Below. CT Staging: T4N2M0

Clinical details: A 65-year-old female presented with an acute episode of PR bleeding, and colonoscopy found a mass lesion in the splenic flexure. Histology confirmed moderately differentiated adenocarcinoma. Patient proceeded with neoadjuvant chemotherapy.

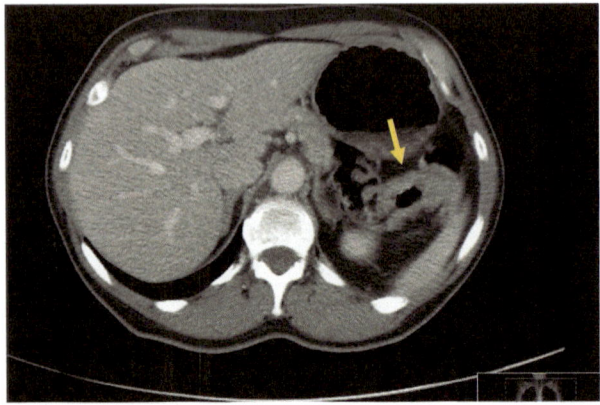

Teaching points: CT scan is the primary imaging modality for staging colon cancer, alongside colonoscopy. It is very useful to delineate the extent of colon primary and to assess its relationship with adjacent organs or structures as illustrated in this case.

7.4 Case 4: An Approximately 5 cm Annular Adenocarcinoma Within the Sigmoid Colon with Peri-colonic Extramural Infiltration. CT Staging: T3N1M0

Clinical details: An 83-year-old male presented with lower abdominal pain and bowel obstruction. Histology confirmed moderately differentiated adenocarcinoma (Fig. 7.1).

Teaching points: CT scan is the primary imaging modality for staging colon cancer, alongside colonoscopy. It is very useful to delineate the extent of colon primary and to assess its relationship with adjacent organs, and, in addition to trans-axial images, reviewing the lesion using all three dimensions provides useful information as illustrated in this case.

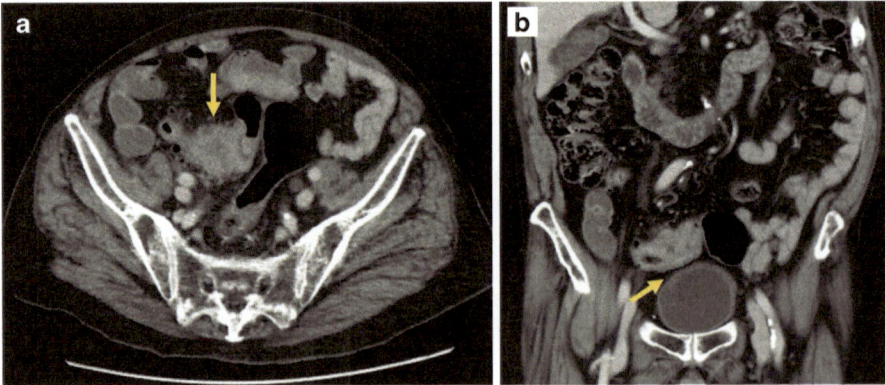

Fig. 7.1 (**a**) Transaxial image of CT scan demonstrates the approximately 5 cm annular mass in the sigmoid colon with extramural infiltration; (**b**) coronal image of CT scan in the same patient demonstrates the clear separation between the tumour and the bladder. Patient proceeded to surgery

7.5   Case 5: Caecum Primary with Mesenteric Nodal and Extensive Liver Metastases. CT Staging: T3N1M1

Clinical details: An 88-year-old female presented with weight loss and microcytic anaemia. Histology confirmed poorly differentiated adenocarcinoma. Patient was recommended for palliative care (Fig. 7.2).

Teaching points: CT scan is the primary imaging modality for staging colon cancer, alongside colonoscopy. It is very useful to delineate the extent of colon primary and detecting metastases as illustrated in this case.

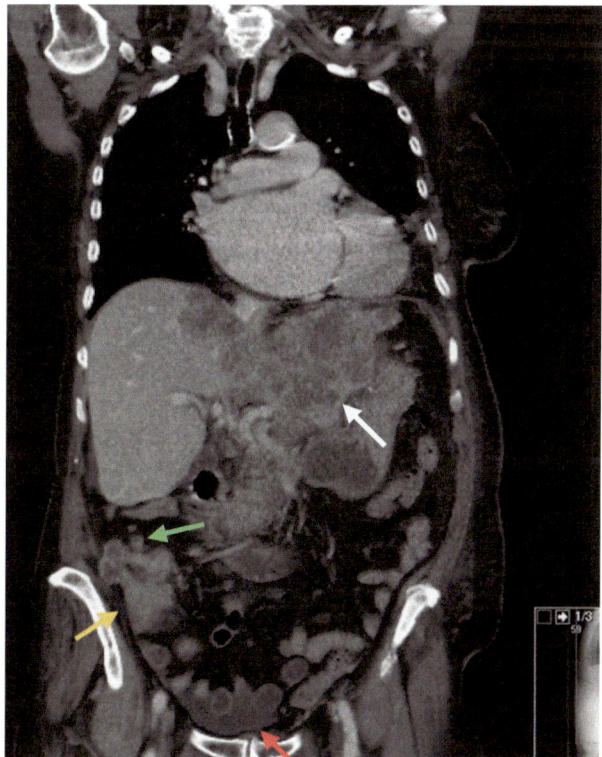

Fig. 7.2 Coronal image of CT scan demonstrates the approximately 5 cm annular mass in the caecum (*yellow arrowed*) with locoregional nodal metastases (*green arrowed*) and large liver metastases (*white arrowed*) and small volume ascites (*red arrowed*)

7.6   Case 6: An Approximately 4 cm Annular Adenocarcinoma Within the Descending Colon with Peri-colonic Nodal Metastases and Adjacent Peritoneal Infiltration. CT Staging: T4N2M0

Clinical details: A 69-year-old male presented with PR bleeding, and colonoscopy found a necrotic mass lesion in the descending colon. Histology confirmed moderately differentiated adenocarcinoma. CT scan demonstrated an approximately 4 cm annular mass in the descending colon with locoregional nodal metastases (Fig. 7.3) and infiltration to the adjacent peritoneum (Fig. 7.3b). Patient proceeded to surgery.

Teaching points: CT scan is the primary imaging modality for staging colon cancer, alongside colonoscopy. It is very useful to delineate the extent of colon primary and to assess its relationship with adjacent organs or structures as illustrated in this case.

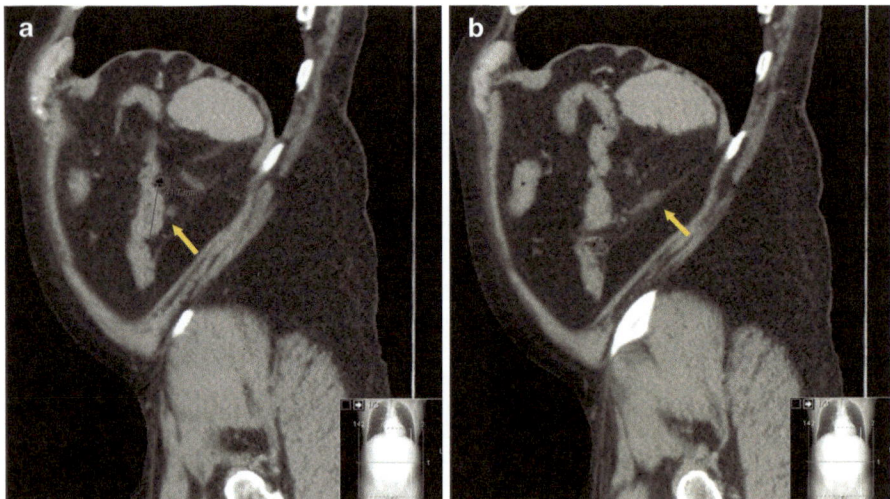

Fig. 7.3 (**a**) Sagittal image of CT scan demonstrates the colon primary in the descending colon as well as an adjacent nodal metastasis; (**b**) sagittal image of CT scan in the same patient demonstrates peritoneal thickening, posterior to the colon primary, consistent with disease infiltration and thus T4 disease

7.7   Case 7: An Approximately 5 cm Annular Adenocarcinoma Within the Transverse Colon in a Patient with a History of Chronic Lymphocytic Leukaemia (CLL). CT Staging: T3N1M0

Clinical details: An 81-year-old female with a history of CLL for 14 years presented with diarrhoea, thought to be related to chemotherapy for her CLL. Colonoscopy found an annular mass lesion in the transverse colon. Histology confirmed poorly differentiated adenocarcinoma. CT scan demonstrated an approximately 5 cm annular mass in the transverse colon with widespread generalised lymphadenopathy above and below the diaphragm (Fig. 7.4).

Teaching points: CT scan is the primary imaging modality for staging colon cancer, alongside colonoscopy. It is however sometimes difficult to differentiate metastatic lymphadenopathy from underlying haematological proliferative disorders such as low-grade lymphoma or CLL, as illustrated in this case.

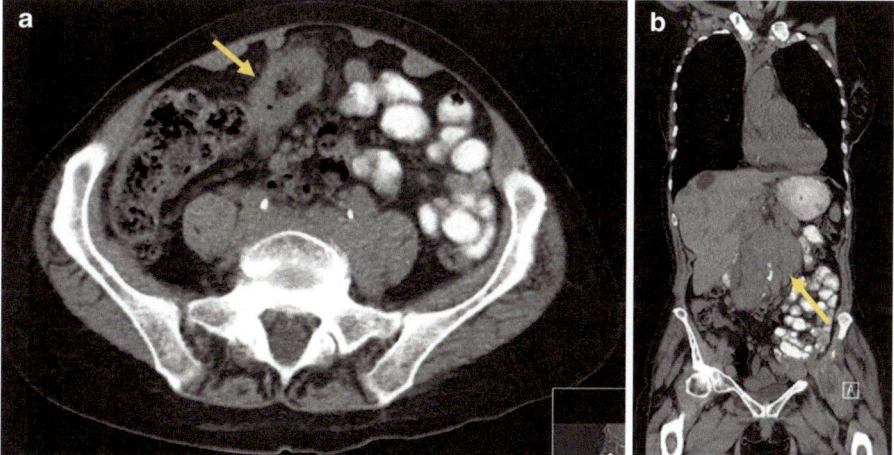

Fig. 7.4 (**a**) CT scan demonstrates the transverse colon primary as well as small volume mesenteric nodes; (**b**) coronal image of CT scan in the same patient demonstrates widespread lymphadenopathy

7.8   Case 8: An Approximately 2 cm Semi-annular Adenocarcinoma Within the Rectum. MRI Staging: T2N0M0

Clinical details: A 78-year-old male with known prostate cancer. MRI for prostate found an incidental rectal tumour. Histology confirmed moderately differentiated adenocarcinoma. MRI scan demonstrated an approximately 2 cm semi-annular mass confined to the 2–5 o'clock position as illustrated below.

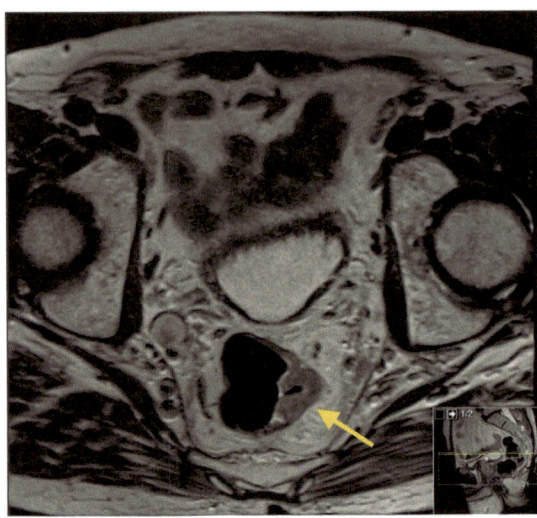

Teaching points: MRI scan is the primary imaging modality for assessing rectal cancer. It is very useful to delineate the extent of rectal primary and to assess its relationship with adjacent musculature and thus guide surgery.

7.9   Case 9: Moderately Differentiated Adenocarcinoma of the Low Rectum. MRI Staging: T4N2M0

Clinical details: A 31-year-old male presented with a history of rectal bleeding, and flexible sigmoidoscopy showed low rectal cancer extending into the anal canal. MRI scan below demonstrates an annular tumour with extramural spread anteriorly at 1 o'clock position and contacts the posterior surface of the prostate gland.

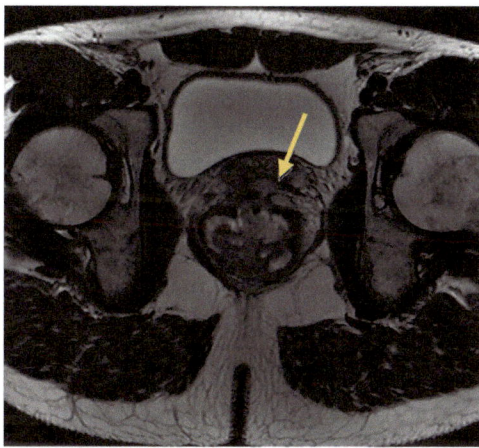

Teaching points: MRI scan is the primary imaging modality for assessing rectal cancer. It is very useful to delineate the extent of rectal primary and to assess its relationship with adjacent musculature and organs and thus guide the management.

7.10   Case 10: Locally Advanced Adenocarcinoma Within the Rectum Extending for Approximately 7 cm in Craniocaudal Length. MRI Staging: T4N2Mx

Clinical details: A 32-year-old male presented with increased bowel frequency and passing blood. MRI scan demonstrated a locally advanced low rectal tumour with anterior extramural spread and contacts the prostate gland at 9 o'clock as illustrated below. Histology confirmed poorly differentiated adenocarcinoma.

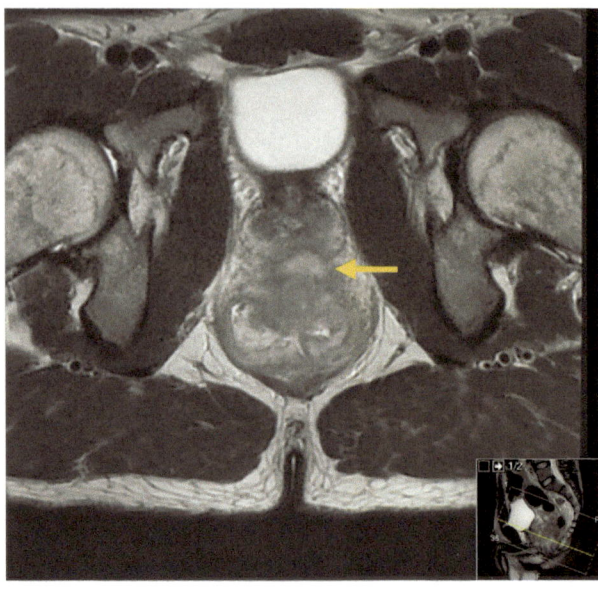

Teaching points: MRI scan is the primary imaging modality for assessing rectal cancer. It is very useful to delineate the extent of rectal primary and to assess its relationship with adjacent musculature and organs and thus guide management.

7.11   Case 11: Locally Advanced Rectal Adenocarcinoma with Multiple Mesorectal Nodal Metastases. FDG-PET/ CT Staging: T4N2M0

Clinical details: A 46-year-old male presented with rectal bleeding. Biopsy confirmed poorly differentiated adenocarcinoma. FDG-PET/CT scan demonstrates metabolically active rectal primary coupled with multiple mesorectal nodal metastases as illustrated below.

Teaching points: FDG-PET/CT scan is a very useful tool in assessing colorectal cancer especially in detecting distant metastases. One of the pitfalls is urinary activity in the pelvis like in this case: the rectal primary is strongly FDG avid, so it is the enlarged right-sided mesorectal nodal metastasis (Fig. 7.5a, b), whilst focal increased FDG accumulation is also seen in the left pelvic region (arrowed) but with no corresponding nodal lesion at this site. This is due to urinary activity in the left ureter as better illustrated in the MIP of the study in Fig. 7.5c.

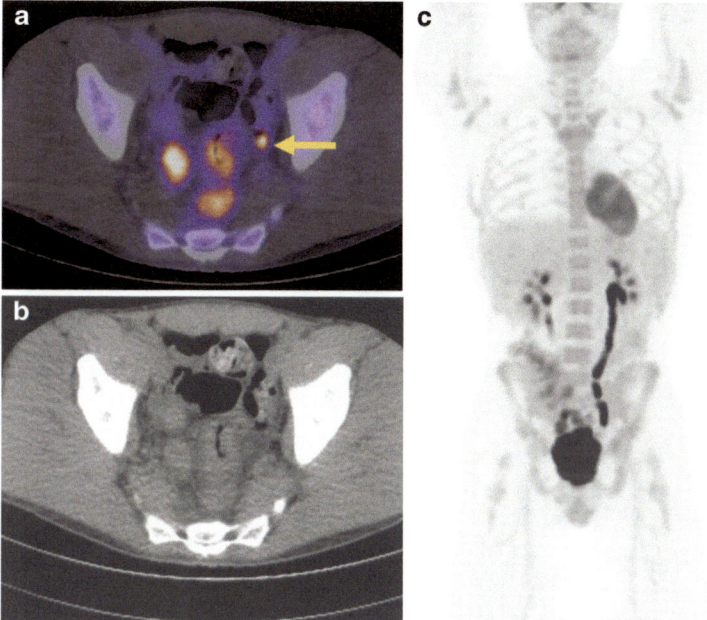

Fig. 7.5

7.12   Case 12: Moderately Differentiated Transverse Colon Cancer with a Solitary Segment VIII Liver Metastasis on Staging CT Scan and Subsequent Liver MRI Scan Was Indeterminate. FDG-PET/CT Staging: T3N1M0

Clinical details: A 71-year-old male presented with anaemia, and colonoscopy confirmed moderately differentiated adenocarcinoma of the transverse colon. The staging CT scan demonstrated T3 N1 transverse primary with a solitary liver metastasis (Fig. 7.6a, arrowed) which was further assessed with a dedicated liver MRI, but this lesion was considered as indeterminate (Fig. 7.6b, arrowed). Subsequent FDG-PET/CT scan demonstrated FDG-avid colon primary (Fig. 7.6c, arrowed), but the concerned liver lesion showed no increased metabolic activity, likely to be a benign lesion.

Teaching points: FDG-PET/CT scan is a useful tool in assessing colorectal cancer especially in characterising indeterminate lesions detected by CT or MRI, as illustrated in this case.

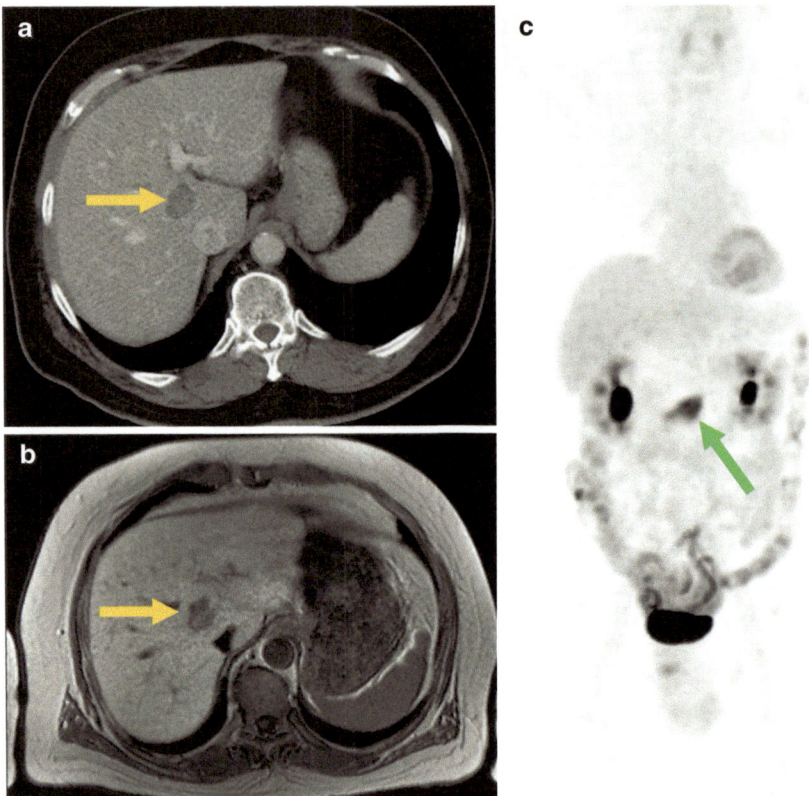

Fig. 7.6

7.13   Case 13: Recurrent Poorly Differentiated Adenocarcinoma of the Rectum 3 Years After Surgery

Clinical details: An 88-year-old male, raising CEA 3 years after anterior resection of rectal primary (T2N0M0 at presentation). FDG-PET/CT scan demonstrates a solitary FDG-avid soft tissue lesion in the right presacral space. Patient proceeded with palliative radiotherapy with subsequent CEA reduction from 15 to 6 (Fig. 7.7).

Teaching points: FDG-PET/CT scan is a very useful tool in detecting recurrent rectal cancer especially in identifying recurrent disease from postsurgical scarring tissue usually in the presacral space as illustrated in the case.

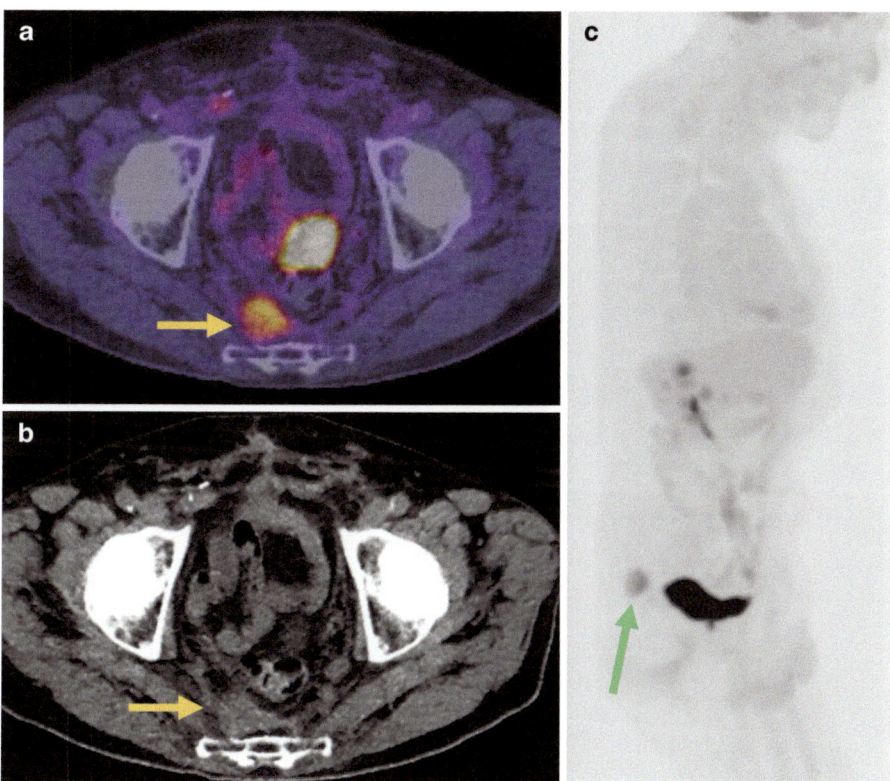

Fig. 7.7 (**a**) Fused FDG-PET/CT scan demonstrates the approximately 2.8 × 23 cm FDG-avid presacral soft tissue (yellow arrowed); the lesions can be identified on the corresponding unenhanced CT image (**b**) (*yellow arrowed*); this lesion is also identifiable in the lateral view of the MIP image (**c**) (*green arrowed*)

7.14   Case 14: Recurrent Colon Cancer 8 Years After Surgery

Clinical details: A 67-year-old female with a history of colon cancer (resected 8 years ago) presented with daily central and lower abdominal pain, frequent loose stools. CEA elevated. CT scan showed new soft tissue thickening along the SMA, suspicious for recurrent disease. FDG-PET/CT demonstrated increased metabolic activity. Patient proceeded with chemotherapy (Fig. 7.8).

   Teaching points: FDG-PET/CT scan is a very useful tool in detecting recurrent colorectal cancer especially in identifying recurrent disease at less usual recurrent sites as illustrated in the case.

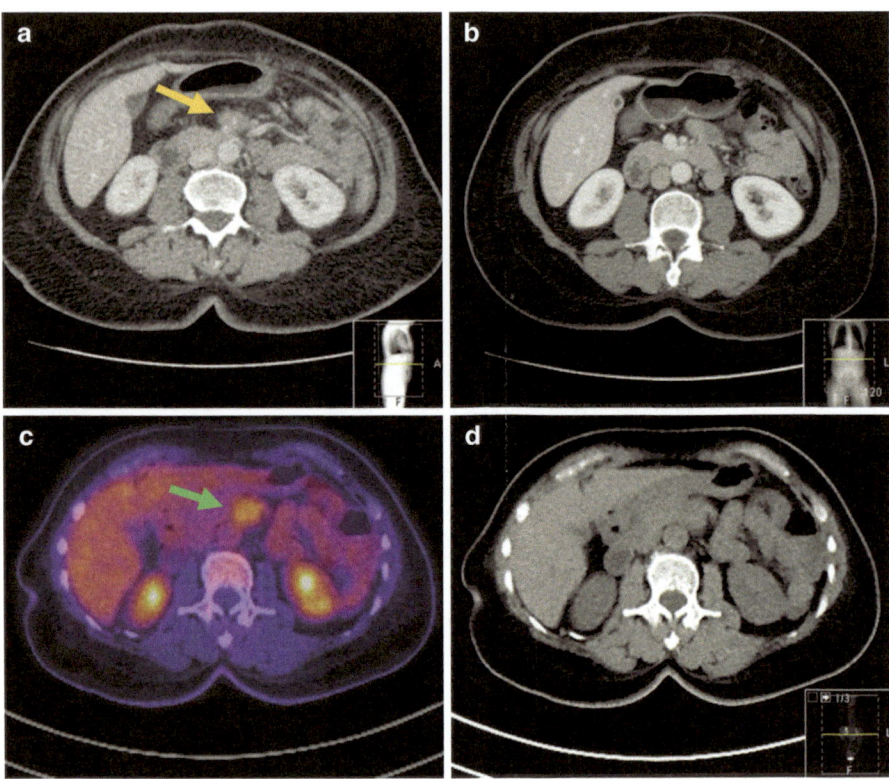

Fig. 7.8 (**a**) CT scan demonstrates soft tissue thickening along the SMA (*yellow arrowed*) which was not present in the previous CT scan 2 years ago (**b**) on subsequent FDG-PET/CT scan (**c**); this soft tissue demonstrates increased metabolic activity (*green arrowed*). (**d**) is the corresponding unenhanced CT image of the FDG-PET/CT study

7.15 Case 15: Further Recurrence in the Right Hilum Following Resection of Solitary Lung Metastasis from a Dukes B Colon Cancer

Clinical details: An 81-year-old female who had anterior resection 3 years ago for a moderately differentiated adenocarcinoma of the sigmoid colon. Had right upper lobectomy a year later for a solitary lung metastasis. Follow-up CT scan 2 years later showed suspicious recurrence in the right hilum. FDG-PET/CT scan demonstrates FDG-avid right hilar soft tissue recurrence. Patient proceeded with cyberknife radiotherapy (Fig. 7.9).

Teaching points: FDG-PET/CT scan is a very useful tool in detecting recurrent colorectal cancer especially in identifying recurrent disease at less usual recurrent sites or postsurgical sites where the normal anatomy was disturbed, as illustrated again in the case.

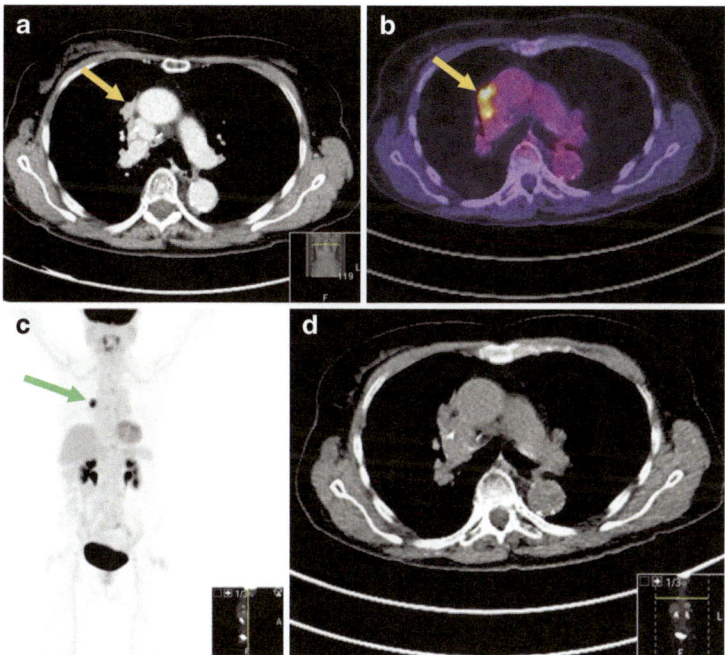

Fig. 7.9 (**a**) CT scan demonstrates soft tissue thickening at the right anterior hilum (*yellow arrowed*) which raised suspicion for further recurrent disease at this site. However, due to the previous surgery, it is less certain if this small soft tissue actually reflects recurrent disease. Subsequent FDG-PET/CT study showed significantly increased metabolic activity, (**b**) fused image, (**c**) MIP and (**d**) unenhanced CT image of the PET/CT study

7.16   Case 16: FDG-PET/CT Has Higher Sensitivity in Detecting Recurrent Colorectal Cancer

Clinical details: A 71-year-old male with a history of sigmoid cancer (resected 3 years ago). Elevated CEA and CT scan showed anastomotic recurrence as well as pelvic nodal metastases. FDG-PET/CT scan demonstrates, in addition, small but FDG-avid extra-pelvic left para-aortic nodal metastases, and as a result, the patient became ineligible for radiotherapy (Fig. 7.10).

   Teaching points: FDG-PET/CT scan has higher specificity and also higher sensitivity in detecting recurrent colorectal cancer as illustrated in the case.

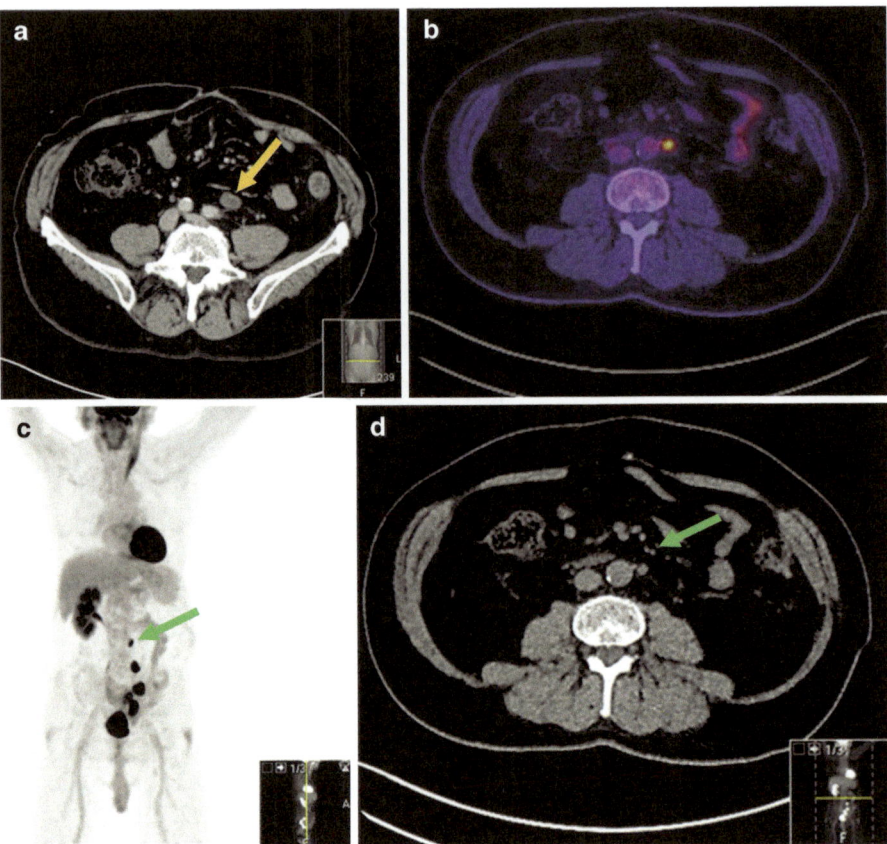

Fig. 7.10 (**a**) CT scan demonstrates anastomotic and other pelvic recurrent lesions including the left common iliac nodal metastasis/recurrence as illustrated in this figure (*yellow arrowed*), but subsequent FDG-PET/CT scan showed a further small extra-pelvic approximately 7 mm left para-aortic nodal metastasis at the level of L3 (*green arrowed*) (**b–d**)

7.17 Case 17: Mucinous Colorectal Tumour Has Low FDG Avidity

Clinical details: A 46-year-old male presented with a mucinous adenocarcinoma of the rectum (T3N2M0) 4 years ago, had chemoradiation and is considered for pelvic exenteration surgery. Restaging CT scan showed a new presacral mass with bony destruction (Fig. 7.11a, yellow arrowed), which raised suspicion of disease infiltration, but this is complicated by the recent chemoradiation. On subsequent FDG-PET/CT scan, this mass demonstrates only very low-grade FDG avidity (Fig. 7.11b, green arrowed). Biopsy confirmed mucinous adenocarcinoma.

    Teaching points: Mucinous colorectal adenocarcinoma is known to have low FDG avidity, and thus FDG-PET/CT scans should be interpreted with caution.

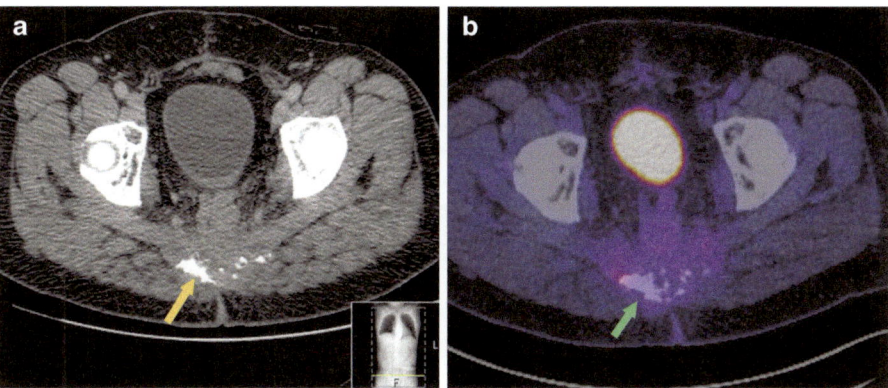

Fig. 7.11

7.18   Case 18: Postsurgical Inflammatory Changes Could Remain FDG Avid for a Protracted Time

Clinical details: A 40-year-old male with recurrent adenocarcinoma of the rectum (anastomotic recurrence 4 years after anterior resection). In addition to the known peri-anastomotic recurrence (Fig. 7.12c, green arrowed), the FDG-PET/CT scan also showed an ill-defined area of FDG-avid soft tissue thickening in the left breast (yellow arrowed in Fig. 7.12a–c) which actually corresponds to a port-a-cath removal 9 weeks prior to the PET/CT scan.

Teaching points: Postsurgical inflammatory changes could remain FDG avid for a protracted time. It is always important to correlate imaging findings with clinical information especially when "unusual" findings are seen as illustrated in this case, whereas a left breast "lesion" was seen in a male patient.

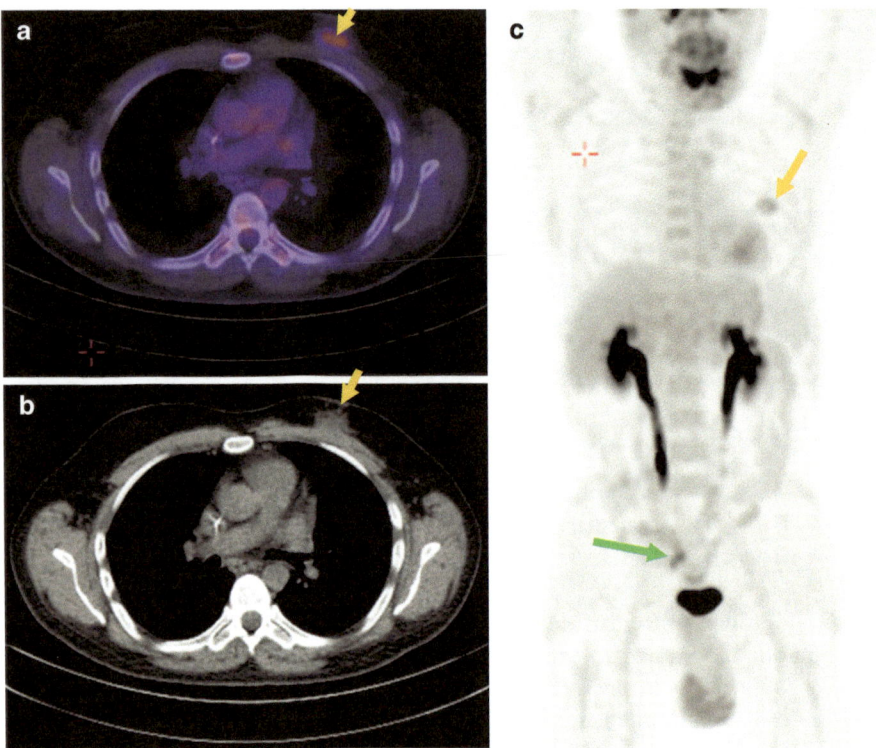

Fig. 7.12

7.19 Case 19: MRI in Assessing Response to Neoadjuvant Chemoradiotherapy in Lower Rectal Cancer

Clinical details: A 48-year-old male presented with rectal bleeding, and biopsy demonstrated moderately differentiated adenocarcinoma of the lower rectum. MDT recommended chemoradiation (Fig. 7.13).

Teaching points: Differing from that of colon cancer, neoadjuvant chemoradiation plays instrumental roles in the treatment of lower rectal cancer. Although no imaging could predict a definite pathological complete remission, both MRI and FDG-PET/CT provide reliable information in assessing response to treatment.

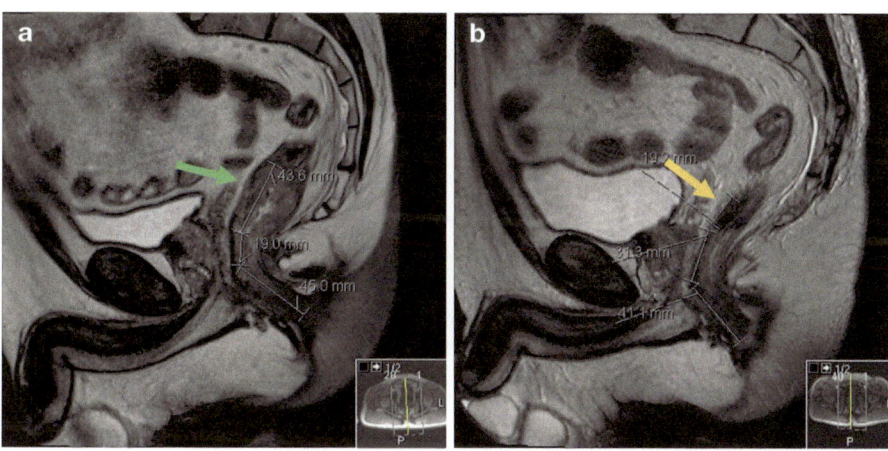

Fig. 7.13 (**a**) Sagittal view of the baseline pelvic MRI scan demonstrates an approximately 4.4 cm annular mass in the lower rectum with its lower edge approximately 1.9 cm above the top of the puborectalis sling (*green arrowed*, MRI stage: T2N0Mx); (**b**) is the same view taken 8 weeks after the completion of chemoradiation and demonstrates an excellent response to treatment with an approximately 1.9 cm predominantly residual scarring tissue at the primary disease site (*yellow arrowed*)

7.20   Case 20: FDG-PET/CT Is a very Useful Tool in Assessing Colorectal Cancer in Response to Chemo- or Radiotherapy

Clinical details: A 50-year-old male presented with a locally advanced rectosigmoid signet ring cell adenocarcinoma. Baseline FDG-PET/CT scan (Fig. 7.14a) demonstrated a strongly FDG-avid rectosigmoid primary (yellow arrowed) and multiple mesorectal nodal metastases (green arrowed); subsequent FDG-PET/CT scan after chemoradiation demonstrated a partial response at the primary site (Fig. 7.14b, yellow arrowed), whilst the previous FDG-avid nodal metastases had mostly resolved.

Teaching points: FDG-PET/CT scan is a very useful tool in assessing colorectal cancer response to treatment. Although low-grade residual FDG uptake could represent either small residual active tumour or post-treatment inflammatory process, focal, high-grade uptake usually reflects residual active disease as illustrated in this case. Also, despite some of the mucinous and signet ring cell adenocarcinomas

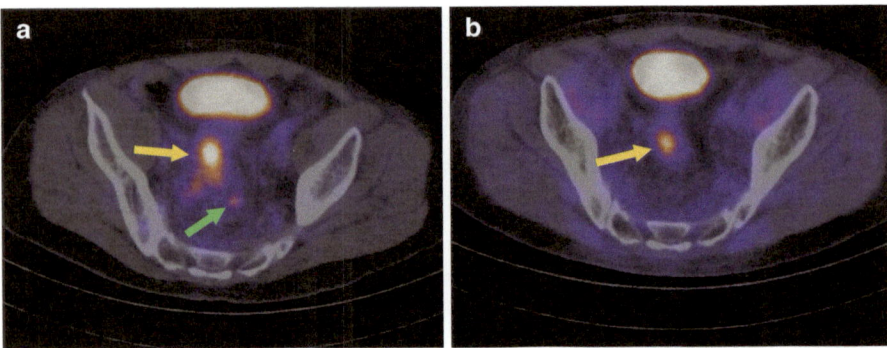

Fig. 7.14

could demonstrate only very low-grade FDG avidity, this is highly variable sometimes depending on the tumour cellularity and mucin content; as shown in this case,
a signet ring cell tumour demonstrates high-grade FDG avidity.

Index

A

Adenocarcinoma, 20
  adjacent peritoneal infiltration, 71–72
  after anterior resection, 77–78
  chemotherapy, 78–79, 84–85
  CLL, 72–73
  craniocaudal length, 74–75
  CT scan, 76–77
  extensive liver metastases, 71
  FDG-PET/CT scan, 80–81
  flexible sigmoidoscopy, 74
  low FDG avidity, 81–82
  mesenteric nodal, 71
  MRI, 73–74, 76–77
  multiple mesorectal nodal metastases,
    75–76
  neoadjuvant chemoradiotherapy, 83–84
  peri-colonic nodal metastases, 71–72
  postsurgical inflammatory changes, 82–83
  radiotherapy, 84–85
  sigmoid colon, 69–71
  solitary lung metastasis, 79–80
  splenic flexure, 69–70
  transverse colon, 68
Adjacent peritoneal infiltration, 71–72
Artefacts
  attenuation correction, 42
  bone lesions, 48–49
  colon and small bowel, 45–47
  liver, 42–44
  lymph nodes, 50–52
  misregistration, 40–42
  muscle metastases/deposits, 48, 50
  normal variants, 62
    diabetic patients, 63
    diverticulitis, 63
    18FDG-PET/CT scanning, timing, 64
    mucinous/signet ring cancer, 63
    non-specific uptake, 63
    presacral mass, 64
    urinary activity, 63
  partial volume effect, 42
  peritoneum, 51–52
  reproductive system, 47
  spleen, pancreas, and adrenals, 44–45
  stomach, 45
  treatment, 53–55
  truncation, 42
  urinary tract, 46, 48
Assessment
  advantages, 32–33
  baseline staging, 32–33
  MRI, 33–35
  response, 61–62
  tumour response, 32

B

Barium enema, 14

C

Carcinoembryonic antigen (CEA), 26
Carcinoid tumours, 20
Chronic lymphocytic leukaemia (CLL),
  72–73
Circumferential resection margin (CRM),
  25, 34
Clinical indications, 60
Colon carcinoma, 15
Colonoscopy, 14
CT colonography, 14–15
Cytotoxics, 26–27

D

Diagnosis, 13, 60–61
Doublet-chemotherapy regimens, 26–27

© Springer International Publishing Switzerland 2017
Y. Du (ed.), *PET/CT in Colorectal Cancer*, Clinicians' Guides to Radionuclide
Hybrid Imaging, DOI 10.1007/978-3-319-54837-1